A Study of Story Telling
Humour and Learning
in Medicine

© Nuffield Trust 2000

Cover Drawing by Mel Calman © S & C Calman

Applications for reproduction should be made to
The Nuffield Trust
59, New Cavendish Street,
London, W1M 7RD

ISBN 011702516X

First published 2000
Second impression 2002

The Nuffield Trust

The Nuffield Trust for research and policy studies in health services was established by Viscount Nuffield in 1940. Today the Trust acts as an independent commentator on the UK health scene and the National Health Service. It has set out to illuminate current issues through informed debate, meetings and publications; and has also commissioned research and policy studies aimed at the development of policy and improvement of health services.

Address:
59 New Cavendish Street,
London
W1M 7RD
UK

Tel: 020 7631 8450
Fax: 020 7631 8451

Email: mail@nuffieldtrust.org.uk
Internet: http://www.nuffieldtrust.org.uk

Printed in the United Kingdom for the Stationery Office

EIGHTH

H.M.QUEEN ELIZABETH THE QUEEN MOTHER FELLOWSHIP

A Study of Story Telling Humour and Learning in Medicine

Kenneth C Calman

THE UNIVERSITY OF DURHAM

FOREWORD BY SIR PETER USTINOV

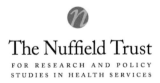

The Nuffield Trust

FOR RESEARCH AND POLICY
STUDIES IN HEALTH SERVICES

London: The Stationery Office

HER MAJESTY QUEEN ELIZABETH THE QUEEN MOTHER FELLOWSHIP

Her Majesty Queen Elizabeth the Queen Mother, who is the Patron of the Trust and has always shown a keen interest in its work, approved the founding of the Fellowship by the Trust to commemorate her 80th birthday.

The Trustees of The Nuffield Trust will select a Fellow who will be invited to undertake a review in a monograph of a subject within the sphere of the Trust which is believed to be of particular interest to Her Majesty. The monograph will be launched by a lecture.

The Nuffield Trust

The Nuffield Trust for research and policy studies in health services was established by Viscount Nuffield in 1940. Today the Trust acts as an independent commentator on the UK health scene and the National Health Service. It has set out to illuminate current issues through informed debate, meetings and publications; and has also commissioned research and policy studies aimed at the development of policy and improvement of health services.

Address;
59 New Cavendish Street,
London
W1M 7RD, UK

Tel: 020 7631 8450
Fax: 020 7631 8451

Email: mail@nuffieldtrust.org.uk
Internet: http://www.nuffieldtrust.org.uk

TO MY MOTHER WHO TOLD ME MY FIRST STORIES

TO MY FATHER WHO SHOWED ME HOW TO LAUGH

TO THEM BOTH FOR BEGINNING MY LEARNING JOURNEY

THE AUTHOR

Professor Sir Kenneth Calman was born on Christmas Day 1941, in Glasgow. After studying medicine and biochemistry in Glasgow he trained as a surgeon with a special interest in vascular and transplantation surgery. After a spell as an MRC Fellow at the Royal Marsden Hospital and Chester Beatty Institute in London, he returned to Glasgow at the age of 32 as the Foundation Professor of Oncology. He remained in that post for ten years developing particular interests in clinical trials, cell biology, education and patient care. He then became Postgraduate Dean and Professor of Postgraduate Medical Education. He then moved to become Chief Medical Officer, first in Scotland and then in England. During that time he developed his interests in education and cancer care. He was a member of the Executive Board of the World Health Organisation and its Chairman between 1998-9. In 1998 he became Vice-Chancellor and Warden of the University of Durham. His outside interests are in literature, cartoons and humour and walking his big black dog.

Contents

Preface

It is a pleasure and an honour to be asked to deliver the Queen Mother Lecture particularly in this her 100th year. The title is my own though for such an important Fellowship I did not wish the lecture and the monograph to be too frivolous, but to reflect the dignity of the practice of medicine. I have therefore tried to make this a scholarly endeavour reflecting the considerable literature already in this area. It is a fascinating topic, the interaction between humour, learning, and storytelling within a medical context. Much more work remains to be done in this area, and the discussion will try to identify some areas for future research. It is a serious subject and therefore worth study and reflection. If this lecture and monograph are able to stimulate some activity in this topic, then perhaps our patients and ourselves will be happier. This book is aimed at doctors and other health professionals who might have an interest in the topics of learning, storytelling and humour.

Improving quality of life remains an important objective for medicine. Happiness is part of this. Healthy people can be miserable and those with serious illness remarkably happy. There should therefore be no indignity for the profession in looking closely at these subjects. It is the same in population terms. Those who do not have all the good things in life are not necessarily unhappy, and those with everything are not always the best pleased. In a previous existence, I once called for the Department of Health to be re-named as the Department of Health and Happiness, as this was our real mission. It was not well received, though I still think that such an objective is at the heart of improving health. Perhaps its time will come.

In the introductory chapter in the book the genesis of the three themes, storytelling, humour, and learning are set out. Perhaps a more personal word at this stage will put these into context. One of my earliest memories, at the age of about six, was being sent to bed at a late hour, having been found reading in the corner of the sitting room. I have always loved books, their feel and their smell. Opening them is always a delight and a pleasure. As an oncologist I found that I was increasingly using stories for teaching and in the management of patients.

Many of the examples in this book therefore have a cancer focus. I also came across, early in my career, a book by T.K.Munro "The Physician as a Man of Letters, Science and Action" which describes many of the varied aspects of the life and work of the doctor. This book, coupled with the essays of Dr John Brown, a physician in Victorian Edinburgh, whose story "Rab and his Friends" I will quote from later in this book, I became enthused with the history of medicine and medical practice. Another important phase in my career was while teaching medical ethics with my colleague Professor Robin Downie. He taught, and continues to teach me, much about an analytical and philosophical approach to medical problems. We began, in our teaching to use poems, plays and books, to illustrate moral problems. This developed into a course on "Literature and Medicine" which became one of the most exciting and formative parts of my career. Finally, as the Chief Medical Officer for England, I had the opportunity to take this initiative further and to be part of a country wide initiative on the arts and health. This resulted in the involvement of the Nuffield Trust and the two Windsor conferences which followed. The end result of this was the setting up of the Centre for the Arts and Humanities in Health and Medicine at the University of Durham.

In the development of this book I should like to express my thanks to my many colleagues at the University of Durham, who have answered my questions, determined my reading lists, and heard me talk endlessly and even preach on the subject. To all of them I am most grateful. The academic environment at Durham lends itself to thinking freely and in the company of like minds. I should also like to thank the librarians (an often forgotten but wonderful profession) at the University of Durham, The Royal Society of Medicine, and the Royal College of Physicians and Surgeons of Glasgow.

I am delighted that Sir Peter Ustinov agreed to write a Foreword to this Monograph. As Chancellor of the University of Durham he has been a friend and mentor, and I can think of no one better to bring the three strands of this book together, storytelling, humour and learning. He is a master of all of them.

Kenneth C Calman.
Durham, April, 2000

Foreword by Sir Peter Ustinov

It is, of course, a great honour to be asked to contribute a foreword to the book of a person one admires and for whom one has the greatest possible affection. The fact that the book was conceived to celebrate the first century of that wonderful lady, the Queen Mother, a supreme example of equilibrium and measure in all things, only serves to make the sense of occasion even more acute.

The book itself is full of personal thoughts into what amounts, from the patient's point of view, to a psychology of the bedside manner and a guide to the breaking of news, both good and bad. It is a remarkable testimony into the workings of a highly analytical mind, which does not flinch from a bold onslaught on the nature of humour and the art of its dissection. As one who frequently uses humour in order to make a point, and does so instinctively, I am frankly terrified by the boldness of Sir Kenneth's approach to a subject which is taboo to most professional entertainers. The vast majority of them regard their craft as a matter of timing, a musical ear, forever instinctive and therefore the antithesis of the world of whys, wherefores and dry equations. Some of them would even commit the ultimate heresy and admit that they never think about how they got their laughs. A few, out of deep-seated professional superstition, would even say bluntly that they would never get the laughs if they thought, and that excessive thought about such matters brings bad luck.

There are, of course, exceptions in the grey area between clinical analysis and unadulterated instinct. In one of the great Hollywood meeting places, the Hillcrest Club, I was privileged, some forty years ago, to observe a table at which all the great comedians of the time were seated: Fred Allen, Jack Benny, Groucho Marx, George Burns and other immortals. Lit from above and swathed in languorous cigar smoke, they looked like a Rembrandt picture of an anatomy lesson before a congress of surgeons. The comedians were as solemn and as static as that.

Suddenly Jack Benny spoke:

> "Let me ask you fellows this: is it funnier, in the story I told you a
> while ago, if the old Jewish lady slips on the banana peel at the top of
> the staircase, and that that is the cause of her falling to the bottom - or
> should she fall first only to slip on the banana peel when she tries to get
> up at the bottom?"

There was a pause of at least thirty seconds, taken up with rumination on the problem. Eventually, George Burns spoke up with his voice of gravel, twirling a wet cigar butt over and over in his mouth:
    "Try it both ways," he suggested.
This seems to be the eternal reaction of the instinct to an attempt at analysis.

In Chapter Four, entitled "Humour", Sir Kenneth boldly attacks the subject from a clinical base, enumerating with rare authority the actual muscles of the face which make laughter in a person apparent to the outside observer. Involved are the muscle groups *zygomaticus major and minor, levator anguli oris, levator labii superioris*, part of the *levator labii superioris alaeque nasi,* and the *risorius* muscle. This is very valuable information, because there was a king in English history, an early Henry or Edward, I forget which, who was reputed never to have smiled again after he lost his son and heir at sea owing to the sinking of the White Ship. For the first time the laymen may realise how many muscles of His Majesty's face fell into disuse, and were probably atrophied, because of the tragedy. Since all the muscles have Latin names, it also raises the question of which muscles a Greek audience used to laugh at the comedies of Aristophanes, since they pre-dated the Romans. A subject worthy of research.

The bedside manner brings many interesting reflections on the fascinating subject of doctor-patient relationships, and the essential collaboration between the two as allies in the same struggle. Naturally Sir Kenneth sees this relationship from the point of view of the medical man, who understands all too well the feelings of a sick person. As such, his opinions are at once compassionate and resolute, relentlessly intelligent and, at times, visionary. I can only comment briefly, as a patient. Throughout my life, there have been determined efforts to remove my gall bladder. Over half a century ago, an elderly surgeon advised me to have the operation,

"But, whatever you do," he pleaded, "don't go to a younger surgeon. I remember all too well...it was my first operation as a fully-fledged professional...and...it might have been nerves, or a moment of aberration...I made an elementary mistake...I won't bore you with the details, but...a corpulent woman it was...died instantly."

He shuddered at the thought. Then suddenly cheered up, and said, "I'll do it for you if you wish."

Recently, a Swiss professor advised me once again to have it out.

"En-est vous sûr?" I asked.

"Monsieur, dans la médicine, on ne peut être sûr de rien!" he replied.

Needless to say I still have my gall bladder.

A charming example of medical tact and understanding is shown in this story from Austria. A very old man goes to the doctor, but seems unwilling to say what is wrong. He looks incessantly at the door. The doctor understands.

"Nurse, please close the door and stay outside until I call you."

Still the old man remains tongue-tied.

"You can speak freely here," he tells the old man.

Eventually the old man speaks.

"Doctor...I am very unhappy...I can only make love on average once a month."

The doctor takes notes.

"But how old are you, sir?" he enquires.

"You'll have to speak a little louder."

"HOW OLD ARE YOU?"

"Eighty-Seven."

"Well, that's remarkable. At your age, I'm suprised you can manage it at all."

"Oh no no." The old man is adamant. "My brother is two years older than I am, and he says he makes love once a week."

The doctor considers this and adds:

"Well...why don't you say the same thing?"

I once wrote that, to arrive at the truth the Germans add, the French subtract and the English change the subject. To find out what the Scots do, I invite you to read this engaging volume.

1. Introduction

"We dream in narrative, daydream in narrative, remember, anticipate, hope, despair, believe, doubt, plan, revise, criticise, construct, gossip, learn, and live by narrative." *Barbara Hardy in "Narrative as a primary act of mind." 1977. In The Cool Web, pp12-33, M. Meek, A. Warlow and G Barton (Eds) London: Bodley Head.*

"We are all learning a respect for narrative as everyone's rock bottom capacity, but also as a universal gift. *Robert Coles in "The call of stories. Teaching and the moral imagination", 1989. Boston: Houghton Mifflin.*

"Narrative is one of the fundamental sense making operations of the mind, and it appears to be both peculiar and universal throughout humanity." *David Lodge in "Narration with words." 1990. In Images and Understanding, H. Barlow, C Blakemore, and M. Weston-Smith (Eds) pp141-153, Cambridge University Press*

"Man lives surrounded by his stories and the stories of others. He sees everything that happens to him through them and he tries to live his life as if he were recounting it." *J P Sarte Nausea 1965, p61 Harmondsworth, England.*

Stories are part of our lives. We live by stories and learn by stories. They are part of our tradition through sagas, fairy stories, ballads and children's stories. We listen to stories from a very early age and they influence our development and thinking. At the other end of life, in our anecdotage, stories, recollections and reminiscences add to our quality of life and to maintaining links with the past and the future. They may be transmitted by mouth verbally, or in written form. More recently they may be conveyed by other means such as film, theatre or television, games or multi-media and the world-wide web. The opportunity to tell and listen to stories grows by the day. Some stories have a universal appeal and others are particular to a specific group or culture.

Within this framework doctors and medical stories have a place, and this book considers medicine as a whole within this very broad range. Doctors are thus no exception in their need to tell and listen to stories and tales. Indeed the basis of this book is that stories are at the heart of clinical practice. This book thus begins by describing what stories are and what their purpose might be. It looks to evidence for their value.

How then did this book have its genesis? First it began with an interest in learning, and a fascination with the way in which some things are easy to learn, others difficult, and the feeling that some people seem to learn more readily than others. This difference could not simply be put down to the level of knowledge, otherwise no one would smoke cigarettes. It had to be more than that. As a medical teacher it was possible to try out new ways of presenting knowledge and facilitating learning, and stimulate enthusiasm and interest in the subject. This provided the impetus to develop an understanding of the ways in which learning occurred.

The second strand was an interest in humour, and particularly in cartoons. These seemed to connect with students and enhance teaching in a remarkably effective fashion, and opened up different ways of considering the same topic and exposing new ways of thinking. It was the interaction between the different contexts which made one laugh. It was clear that this had relevance to learning as the same mechanism, connecting two or more unrelated issues, seemed to operate: a new idea seen in an old context causing a revision of thinking and behaviour. It was at this time that the idea of the contagious theory of behaviour change was conceived. This hypothesis, to be dealt with in several places in the book, but most fully in Chapter 9, suggests that behaviour is caught by the transmission of ideas from one person to another. The agent responsible is the Transmid, a transmitted idea, and this concept will be referred to regularly. While this is not a new thought it did provide a vehicle for the discussion of storytelling (the transmission of ideas) in a different setting, and with a different purpose.

The third strand was the telling of stories. Reading had always been a special pleasure, and the tales created by other writers were able to open up new ways of thinking about the world. It was also relevant that doctors tended to talk in stories (about patients, incidents, experiences) and to learn in stories. These three themes became more visible on the reading of Arthur Koestler's book "The Act of Creation". This gave a unified concept to the three strands, as they were indeed three aspects of the same thing, namely creativity. Stories were a means by which learning could occur, and they did so by changing our way of thinking about a particular topic. Similarly, humour, comedy, wit, and the many other similar words used, allow us to see things in a new light. Finally in the context of curiosity and discovery, artistic creativity, invention and innovation, it is the ability to see something that no one else has recognised and to present it in a form which allows others to discover what was always there. A remarkable process. This then was the beginning of this study.

It was expanded on the reading of Howard Gardner's book, "Leading Minds: An anatomy of leadership". As an educationalist, Gardner had explored the role of storytelling in recognised world leaders. He concluded that good leaders always had a clear story to tell, which others would wish to follow or emulate. The tale was often told as a parable, or was rich in examples and allusions. The Teller did not need to be an orator, or charismatic, but did need to have a powerful tale to relate. This seemed to fit the mould of medical leaders. People who could enthuse, excite, and stimulate thinking and ideas. They were both good teachers, and good research workers; there is a synergy between the two and they are not mutually exclusive. It was also clear that all professions and groups need leaders. Those who have gone before, who have broken the mould, fought the battle and won, and gained the golden ring, are a very special group. Such tales about leadership abound in the literature and are well captured in Joseph Campbell's book, "A Hero With a Thousand Faces." Put a few doctors together and soon they are exchanging stories about those with whom they worked and learned from. It is a sort of a way of recognising not only the exploits and feats of others, but of bringing ordinary mortals into the same group. It is an expression of belonging.

These three writers, Koestler, Gardner and Campbell, thus sit at the heart of this book. They have moulded it and shaped it, though the author has met none of them. Such is the power of writing and stories. It is possible to be connected to another person, their ideas and thoughts, through the media of the written or spoken word, even though no personal contact has been made.

Stories may be of all sorts. They may be serious, happy, sad, exciting, depressing and humourous. They may carry messages and have a moral dimension, and may be used to set values and beliefs. Some concentrate on the characters in the story (the patient) and it is this feature which is memorable. Others focus on the theme (the illness) or the message (the lessons). Some may be short or long, and may be simple or complex in consultation. Some people are very good at telling stories or "spinning a yarn", and develop a reputation for this. Others find it more difficult to recount a tale, but can learn to present more effectively. Regularly presenting material on ward rounds and at seminars can be one way of getting the practice and is an important skill.

The language of stories is also important. How ideas are expressed and the pictures that are conjured up are part of this as they stimulate the imagination. This is particularly relevant in the description of illness and, for example, the way in which patients are described, or words which they use to describe themselves. Words such as "victim" and "battle" are regularly used. Susan Sontag in her book "Illness as a Metaphor" (1991) describes some of the problems of language and the way in which it can, and is, used to place people in a particular category. It is surprising how rapidly things can change. One moment you are a healthy human being and the next, because of a few words telling you that you have an illness, you become a patient and enter a different state, with different expectations and emotions. The language is thus critical as it sets the tone and context of the story. Try telling a well known story, pick any fairy tale such as the Three Bears, and change the language to that of the doctor (using anatomical allusions) or the general (with military terms) or the architect (with building terminology) and see the difference.

Stories are thus an important aspect both of communication and the process of learning. Listening is a crucial part of story telling. If no one listens, the story is unheard and has no meaning. An audience is essential, and the interaction between the two is so important, hence its central part in the clinical consultation. This is relevant even if the story is a written one, and concerns subjects which might be considered serious, and even factual. With the written word the presence of the author is always there as the interpreter and narrator of the story. How we learn communication skills is an important question and a great deal of work is currently going on in this area. It is important however to recognise that communication is a value as well as a skill. Talking with patients, and listening to them, is something that every doctor must consider to be important, not a box to be ticked in a curriculum list. A one-week course on how to "communicate" will be irrelevant if it is not seen as something which is an integral part of clinical practice. In particular senior staff must provide the role models and support for juniors and show by example its relevance and importance.

Medical stories and humour are sub-sets of story telling, and this book will look at both of these and consider how they link to education and learning. The relationship between the anecdote and the evidence base will be considered, and the need to connect the individual case history with the world literature. Questions such as "Is this patient's problem unique? What is the best way of managing the problem? Can my experience be related to what others do?" need to be answered. This is not a reaction against the evidence based approach to clinical practice but reflects a different and complementary way of learning and thinking. This concept will be explored later in the book.

It is also about clinical and medical research and the need for curiosity and discovery. Stories allow us to explore areas which are tentative, uncertain, and even heretical. In a safe way we can express new and different ideas, and test them. Listening to patients gives us the text for the research work and they give us the insights sometimes required to see things differently. Incidents in clinical practice, remarks patients make, unusual responses to treatment, all provide possible ways in which new ideas may be generated.

Many stories contain moral lessons and can be used to illustrate ethical issues. They illustrate good and bad, (at least according to the author) and leave the gray areas for debate. Much of clinical work deals with issues of uncertainty and judgement. The use of stories can be one way of raising difficult issues and of exploring the ethical issues in clinical practice.

The history of stories is the history of ideas and of cultures and nations. Stories can last for thousands of years, and be transmitted from generation to generation with great fidelity. In Iran the story tellers are still telling about the exploits of Alexander the Great as if they had just happened. The great stories of the past in the Bible, Chaucer, Shakespeare, Dickens, Scott, Stevenson and many others show how powerful and effective they can be. One of the major questions to be discussed therefore is why some stories are seen to be important and last for a very long time, and others not?

Some stories have a very deep psychological significance and recur again and again in different cultures. They seem to have emerged independently at different times and places. As an example, the meaning and relevance of fairy stories have been analysed in Bruno Bettelheim's book "The Uses of Enchantment." (1976). This is a fascinating account of well known stories and raises many of the concepts first set out by Freud. Fantasy, the pleasure principle, integration, achieving autonomy are all discussed with reference to "The Three Little Pigs", "Little Red Riding Hood", "The Goose Girl" and many others. While this book might just stop you reading such stories to your children, it does raise some fascinating issues, and makes it clear that stories are a most powerful way of maintaining and sustaining a culture.

There is also an important relationship between oral and written stories. In general, oral stories have attracted less attention, and perhaps less credence, than the written word. Folk tales, fairy stories and of course patient stories are very important in preserving standards and culture of any group. The writing down of the story freezes it at a particular point in time and misses the associated non-verbal cues. The feelings of emotion such as anger and fear are less readily communicated in written form than by the oral route. The "performance" associated with telling a tale sets the context and the atmosphere and is an important part of the process. Hearing a real person tell a real story can be a very powerful experience. In a similar way, non verbal stories can be used to explore different views of the world. Our body language and the signals we send out are also powerful stories. Mime and dance can tell much about the human condition and the emotions and feeling we all have.

There is an assumption which runs through some contemporary medical thinking that science is the only basis of clinical practice. There is a feeling that the arts and humanities are less important and don't contribute much in the care of patients. On the other side there are those who see science as the force which removes autonomy and which dictates what patients need, and removes choice and dignity. Of course both are right and the artificial distinction between the two, and the divide which is created, is neither helpful nor productive. Medicine is both an art and a science and it is legitimate to study and to be involved with both. The argument, however, is an old one, and is well described in an article by Tauber (Tauber, 1992). He looks again at the Osler-Flexner debate which began in the early part of the 20th Century. Flexner had visited many of the European medical schools and prepared a Report for the Johns Hopkins Medical School. It advocated a strong science base for medicine. Osler, by now in Oxford, put forward the alternative and emphasised the role of the humanities. The debate continues, but in a sense it is a sterile one. It is reminiscent of C.P.Snow's "The Two Cultures", which highlighted the same issue, but in another context. Having written on both science and the arts (see Calman and Downie, 1996) they must be seen as complementary. This book is a mixture of both.

In a previous book (Calman, 1998) reference was made to the potential for improving health. We already have much of the knowledge we need to improve health, but one of the problems is that we have not put it into practice. Research is vital, we need to know more, but we also need to find ways of making people change. This reference is directed not just to the public to stop smoking, to eat a more balanced diet, and to take more exercise. It is a reference to the need for professionals of all disciplines to consider how they can change the way in which they practice. More than ever they are under scrutiny and more than ever they will need to show that they are implementing the evidence base which is now so publicly available. Stories and a greater understanding of how we learn can contribute to this.

This book therefore explores some of these concepts and ideas related to tales and how they can contribute to improving clinical practice. In addition it discusses the ways in which stories can be used to transmit, not only information, but changes in behaviour. It introduces a new concept, that of the Transmid, a transmitted idea. This contagious theory of behaviour change provides a new way of thinking about how ideas can be disseminated. Humour forms part of this review and its links to learning are also discussed.

So if that is what the book is about, what does it not cover? Much has already been written about narrative in medicine, about humour, and about doctors as storytellers. Doctors in literature as a topic is also well reviewed and will not be covered again in this volume (Calman,1997, Ceccio, 1978, Hunter et al, Jones, 1996, 1995, Lancet,1999, McLellan, 1996, Moore, 1977, Munro,1951). For this reason the reader is referred to such texts for this aspect of the subject. Instead, this book will explore some other aspects of medical writing including the role of textbooks, aphorisms and the newer forms of communication such as the Internet. The topic of medical students in the literature has been less well reviewed and there will therefore be a section on this subject.

It begins, therefore, with a review of storytelling, and considers the purpose of stories and how we understand them. It next looks at humour, and in particular medical humour. The third main topic, that of the mechanism of learning, is the next to be considered. The remainder of the book builds on these three basic areas and subsequent chapters cover other types of stories, medical stories, ethical issues, and the contagious theory of behaviour change.

During the writing of this book there was a brief holiday interlude. It was used as would seem appropriate to "improve each shining hour", by re-reading some classic tales in prose and verse. While they support the thrust of the book, and its conclusions, the section has been placed as an Annexe (Annexe 1) to ensure that the main themes of the book are set out clearly. The reader may wish to consult this Annexe for additional material.

In summary the objectives of this book are to explore the relationship between storytelling, learning and humour, and to try to identify any common threads. It will look at new ways of changing behaviour, using stories, and set out some of the areas of research which still need to be considered. Above all, its aim is to interest the reader in the fascinating issues of storytelling and the link they make to human experience and the quality of all our lives.

REFERENCES

Bettelheim, B. The Uses of Enchantment. 1976. Penguin. Harmondsworth, England.

Calman,K.C. Literature in the education of the doctor. Lancet 1997, 350, 1622-24

Calman, K.C. The Potential for Health. 1998, Oxford University Press.

Calman,K.C. and Downie, R.S. Why arts courses for medical curricula? 1996. Lancet, 347, 1499-50.

Campbell, J. A Hero With a Thousand Faces. 1949. Princeton University Press.

Ceccio,J. Medicine in Literature, 1978. Longman, Inc. New York.

Gardner,H. Leading Minds. An Anatomy of Leadership. 1995. Harper Collins, London

Hunter,K, Charon, R, Coulehan,J.L. The study of literature in medical education. 1995.Academic Medicine. 70, 787-94.

Jones.A.H, Literature and medicine: an evolving cannon. 1996. Lancet, 348, 1360-62

Koestler, A. The Act of Creation. 1964, Hutchison and Co, London

Lancet, Literature and ageing,1999. Lancet supplement III, 354, 1-40

McLellan,F.M. Literature and medicine: some major works. 1996. Lancet,348, 1014-16.

Moore, A.R. Medical Humanities: an aid to ethical discussions. 1977. J.Med.Ethics.3, 26-37.

Munro, T.K. The Physician as a Man of Letters, Science and Action.1951, E and S Livingstone, 2nd Edition, Edinburgh and London

Snow,C.P. The Two Cultures. 1998. Cambridge University Press

Sontag, S. Illness as a Metaphor. 1991. Penguin, Harmondsworth, England

Tauber, A.I. The two faces of medical education: Flexner and Osler re-visited. 1992. Journal of the Royal Society of Medicine. 85, 598-602.

2. The Purpose of Stories

"He remembered how at birth he had put the child at the bottom of the bed, a parcel of useless flesh. It was Mrs Ritchie who had skelped him into life. She would talk about that and it would swell in the telling, it would become a story of a life stolen from the jaws of death." *William McIlvanney in* *"Docherty"*

Introduction

At one level stories can merely amuse, enthral or entertain, at another many can educate and change behaviour. Stories have been used for generations as vehicles for passing on information and wisdom. They can be factual and true, or imagined events, or magical and mysterious and set in other worlds and with strange mystical beings such as fairies and giants. They can stimulate the imagination and excite our curiosity. They can tell moral tales and impart a sense of right and wrong. Stories, however, do have a range of purposes which can be seen both from a medical and a non-medical perspective. This chapter opens up some of the themes which will be developed in later chapters.

1. **To Provide a Framework for Life.** In this sense stories help us to make sense of the world around us. They help us to place ourselves in someone else's shoes, to understand their problems and difficulties and to realise that it is possible to go through a particular problem or life event and come out at the other end. Initiation ceremonies whether in a tribe in some remote part of the world, or as a house officer, fulfil the same function. Someone has been there before and survived to tell the tale.

   Stories create a culture and an environment which, in some circumstances, help to define a group. They provide a hidden agenda within which we operate. Professional groups, such as doctors, often have particularly powerful stories to reinforce the tribal beliefs. Looking ahead to choices or to future directions, such as in career possibilities, the stories of others can help to make sense of our own lives.

The stories patients tell each other are also important and in a similar way reflect the culmination of wisdom and experience. They can be supportive and pass on the reflections of the disease or treatment. The stories patients tell doctors and other health care workers also help to make sense of the professional's life. Why are we doctors? What is the purpose of our healing role? Patients help us to identify our purpose and as we re-tell their stories to others, so we become part of the story itself. Mrs Ritchie, as illustrated in the quotation at the start of this chapter, shows how important that involvement can be.

2. **Dealing With Major Life Events.** This is a subset of the first point, providing a framework for life stories can help us deal with major life events; births; deaths; serious illness; failures. To know that one is not alone, that others have been there before you, is often comforting and valuable. People's stories of how they have dealt with illness, of how doctors have worked day and night to save a child or a mother, of how acts of kindness and dedication can make the difference, all illustrate the power of the story.

Paul Tournier (1982) in his book "Creative Suffering" puts forward the hypothesis that suffering occurs to all of us but what matters is how we deal with it. Doctors, he argues, have two roles, the first to deal with the acute problem presented by the patient, the second to help the patient benefit from the illness. Say that to a patient with a newly diagnosed cancer and you might be surprised at the response. Patients do change when serious illness occurs, and it can be of real benefit.

For the newly qualified doctor dealing with their first death or major illness in a young patient, or an operation which does not go as planned, can be frightening and difficult to deal with. Talking to others, listening to the stories of others, can be comforting and helpful. It will not take away the pain, that will have to be borne personally, but it will ease the concern and anxiety. These rites of passage are part of all cultures, and the medical profession is no exception.

3. **The Therapeutic Effect of Story Telling.** To tell someone your own story has been known for generations as being therapeutic. An attentive listener to whom you can divulge problems and concerns is generally helpful. In all branches of medicine listening to patients and their families is an integral part of the work of the doctor. Much of general practice is about listening to patients

telling their stories. No one should belittle such work. It is integral to the process of the consultation, the building block of the whole health care system. It enables trust to be built up and established. Indeed it is fundamental to the therapeutic relationship. Sometimes the response required is entirely non-directive, no interpretation is required. At other times people seek advice and a direction. The skill of the general practitioner is to know what is required in which patient.

Writing down your story is an extension of this process, sometimes called "Creative Writing" (Bolton 1999). The act of setting down in black and white what you feel, what the problems are, what the good things have been, can be most helpful both for patients and doctors. It can allow subsequent reflection on the story – the tale for the day – and assist in the way in which problems are dealt with. Such written stories make important documents for analysis and interpretation.

In the evening at the end of the day it is good to be able to share with someone else the problems, the burdens, the excitements and discoveries, and the funny things and the sad things. Those who are lonely and lack that opportunity recognise only too well what is missing in their lives. Everyone needs someone to talk to. The art of conversation remains important. The ability to talk and converse about a range of subjects, not just one's own boring interests, to make others feel that they are being listened to, is one of the hallmarks of a civilised society. R.S.Peters, in his book "Ethics and Education" (1966) makes the process of conversation one of the outcomes of education and an attribute of the educated person.

4. **Stories As Records of Events – History.** When stories are collected together over a period of time they provide a history by which the interpretation of events can be seen in context. Traditionally one might think of this in terms of countries, people, places or conflicts. In medical terms the recording of events and of people is often fundamental in understanding the nature of disease and the introduction of treatment. They add a dimension to the practice of medicine which provides us with heroes and legends and gives inspiration for the future. Putting a patient history together over a long period of time may be the only way to solve the problem. This argues against episodic care, and for a long term relationship with the patient and the family.

Histories can be written in different ways and with quite different perspectives. Such differences in interpretation and outlook can be very significant and illustrate some of the problems in getting new stories (ideas) accepted. They also illustrate clearly how the thoughts and ideas of a particular generation of doctors set the paradigms for treatment and care. With hindsight they seem quaint, old fashioned and often quite wrong. It is thus salutary to think that in a generation from now our high technology medicine is likely to appear crude and unsophisticated. As an example, the diagnosis and classification of disease and illness has changed significantly over the years. Indeed it might be said that the whole history of medicine is the re-classification of ideas and of diseases. Take, for example, the history of our thinking on infectious disease, or of cancer. Over the centuries we have called tumours by different names and related them to different causes, and treated them in radically different ways. There is no doubt that in 50 or 100 years our current hypotheses will appear strange and naive.

History is sometimes seen as a way of predicting the future. Understanding the past can help assess the way forward. Not all of course would agree with this, though in clinical terms it is the bread and butter of medical practice. It's called the prognosis. People want to know what will happen to them as a result of disease or injury. Doctors listen to the stories, and supplemented by a few tests, regularly give a view as to what might happen. These are of course probabilities, based on listening to many similar stories. In population terms it is generally possible, but for the individual, much less easy. Soothsaying is part of the doctor's role, though it is our job to refine and improve the predictive component of the task.

Finally there are the histories of famous medical women and men. These, for the reasons given above, can be very illuminating and give insights into the problems faced and the solutions developed. The history of medicine is fascinating and a necessary part of the study of medicine.

5. **Stories As Ways of Assisting Communication.** Communication with people is at the heart of clinical practice. Almost all that doctors do is related to talking to people, breaking bad news, discussing choices, and reviewing progress. In a similar way patients communicate with doctors through stories (case histories). Such stories are generally fuller and richer when delivered by mouth and associated with non-verbal language than in the dry text of a case record. Computer based history taking and the use of ancillary staff to take histories can

make things faster but they can remove the essence of the story and reduce emotions and feelings to a few words or sentences. It is difficult to record tears or anger on a computer. Hence the importance of linking the story to clinical examination and subsequent investigation of the patient, and thus to the prognosis and treatment options. The history from the patient often dictates the latter.

6. **Bridging Generations and Providing Continuity.** Stories can provide the link between generations. The wisdom of the older person linked to the younger one. The experience of a senior consultant or general practitioner can be of great benefit to the younger member of staff. It provides a feeling of continuity, of continually provided care in a particular setting. The process is of course not all one way, and the elders can learn a great deal from the young warriors. Stories can enliven interest and add depth to a speciality. The wisdom and judgement which is generated come from listening to lots of stories, and assimilating the nuances and the patterns. This can be by-passed or enhanced to some extent by a careful review of the related literature, using the patient problem as the index case and comparing it with other stories in books and journals. This link is essential in any case to ensure that a particular case history fits the pattern.

7. **Setting Standards and Values.** One of the major foundations of stories is to set standards and values. Parables, fables, fairy stories all have as their purpose moral values and the definition of good and bad. The legends and sagas provide for the same sorts of messages. Heroes determine the mind set and behaviour pattern. It is the hero and the legend who have won the prize and slain the dragon and thus set standards for good and evil. Goodies and baddies are just as important in medicine as in the media.

Joseph Campbell in his several books (see "A Hero With a Thousand Faces") makes the point that heroes and legends are part of all societies in all cultures and ages. Such individuals provide the focus for a generation, or generations, of doctors by their great deeds and good works. All cultures need them and to some extent the modern world is re-inventing them. We have heroes in sport, in the media, in the arts, and also in medicine.

Medical heroes are important. The internationally known ones, Lister, Osler, the Hunter brothers, Harvey, are all well recorded and their stories provide a fascinating insight into how legends are born. There are also, however, local heroes: clinicians working in difficult environments, delivering an outstanding service, pioneering new techniques, are just as important. They provide the inspiration for those who come after. They become role models by the tales and legends told by them, or about them. Put a few doctors who trained in the same hospital together and within a few minutes they are reminiscing about people and events: they recreate the legend by telling stories and become part of the legend itself. For this reason, if for no other, the social side of medicine needs to be present to provide a mechanism for such tales to be told and re-told.

Such heroes and legends are fundamental in medical practice. They provide the motivation for others, set examples and standards. They are the "goodies" whose practice needs to be emulated.

8. **Stories and Leadership.** Howard Gardner's book "Leading Minds" (1996) makes the point that good leaders tell good stories. They are able to capture an idea or concept and relate it to people in a way which engages them and motivates them. He uses examples of world leaders and examines the power of their stories. The concept he develops is an important one. As has been described, heroes develop around stories, and legends develop around them. They set the pace, they make the running by the story they tell. Such stories, and leaders, may not all be telling "good" messages, some such stories and leaders are evil and corrupt. But the power of the message is so strong that others will follow. Nor does the storyteller have to be charismatic and/or attractive. If the power of the story is great then others will follow.

   So it is in medical practice. Good leaders tend to be good storytellers. They present difficult material and concepts simply and easily. They can converse, explore, expound, use illustrations and examples which fill out a story and make it exciting and understandable. It follows therefore that good leaders make good teachers, and that teaching is an integral part of leading (Simpson and Calman, 2000).

9. **Learning Through Stories.** It follows logically from this discussion that a great deal of learning takes place through stories, and this will be discussed more fully in chapter 5.

Medical education is no different. Doctors learn through telling stories to each other about patients, problems, other doctors and experiences. Presenting cases to each other in ward rounds or clinical meetings is just another form of telling stories. Indeed the analogy can be taken further in that many of these presentations take place on long winter evenings during which the wise men (usually, but not always, older) interpret the stories and draw from their long experience the lessons that can be learned. The wisdom is shared.

At a more basic level the stories told by patients (histories) provide this same powerful educational experience. In a similar way the stories told by relatives and friends about the care given to patients can be both moving and provocative. "Memories" (Calman,1989) was a short paper which reflected on the feelings and concerns of those who had been cared for in a hospital environment. It showed how small details of care were of great importance to individual patients and families. There was generally little concern about the treatment offered, it was generally felt to be very good, but it may be considerable about the general standard of overall care, communication and sensitivity to particular personal needs. We neglect the messages of such stories at our peril.

Involvement with patient support groups is one mechanism for hearing such stories firsthand or listening to patients outside the confines of the clinic or white coats. Such experiences provide very powerful educational lessons for all health professionals. They allow the doctor to be disarmed without the paraphernalia of the profession and to listen to the patient with sympathy and compassion.

10. **Stories As Repositories of Knowledge and Information.** Stories collected together in books and libraries provide immense repositories of information. Electronically available material enhances this prospect. These are spectacular reference sources. To be able to read and make contact with the information and knowledge in the world literature about a clinical problem is surely a remarkable process and the new technology will make it even easier. It is critical therefore that we use this resource, and this book is not a justification for anecdotal medicine. Far from it, indeed it is the opposite. The story (or the history) sets the scene and particularises the problem to an individual. The doctor's responsibility then is to ensure that this patient benefits from the experience of all similar patients and the learning of all those who have helped to manage them. That is what libraries and databanks are for.

In medical terms stories are often collected together in textbooks which contain the collected experience of one or more people in a particular field of medicine or science. The key to such textbooks is how the stories are told, the sequence of the chapters, the structure, the pedagogy, and the authority of the writers. Textbooks in the 21st Century cannot expect to be completely up-to-date, medical knowledge is moving too fast. However, they can be guide books to the subject, taking the learner through a series of steps from which they can move with more detailed, and in some cases, more up-to-date work. In this sense there is a real need for a textbook, as a hitchhikers guide to a subject, but not as the definitive up to the minute review. There are other methods, such as the use of the Internet, to deal with this.

11. **Stories to Amuse and Entertain.** This may seem to be a less serious aspect of story telling, but it is just as important. In all sorts of ways stories add to our quality of life. In relaxing, in reflecting, in taking us into new places and new thoughts and removing us, in the short term, from the routine of life. They provide one mechanism of escape and can help in coping with problems.

Humourous medical stories are the same. They allow doctors to look at themselves and laugh a little. They help us deal with difficult problems and situations. This aspect will be discussed in more detail in Chapter 4.

SOME CONCLUSIONS

Stories have many purposes, often quite serious and fundamental. They help us make sense of the world and able to bear some of the burdens which we face. They give meaning and structure to our daily lives. In medical terms the same situations hold. Stories are part of medical practice and help us understand patients and their needs more effectively, but only if we listen. They help in the development of trust, a key ingredient in the patient-doctor relationship. Stories invite us to be part of someone else's journey. It is our privilege to be allowed to listen to such stories, and engage with them.

REFERENCES

Bolton, G. The Therapeutic Potential of Creative Writing. 1999. Jessica Kingsley Publishers, London.

Calman, K.C. Memories: a neglected concept in care. 1989, Lancet ii, 1185-6

Campbell. J. A Hero with a Thousand Faces. 1949 Princeton University Press.

Gardner, H. Leading Minds. An anatomy of Leadership. 1995. Harper Collins, London.

McIlvaney,W. Docherty. 1975, Sceptre Books.

Peters, R.S. Ethics and Education. 1966. Allen and Unwin, London.

Tournier, P. Creative Suffering. 1982. Translated by Edwin Hudson. SCM Press, London.

Simpson,J and Calman, K.C. Making and preparing leaders. Medical Education. 2000. 34.211-5.

3. Understanding Stories

"Still, however, you must remember, that the tale told by one friend, and listened to by another, loses half of its charms when committed to paper: and that the narratives to which you have attended with interest, as heard from the voice of him to whom they have occurred, will appear less deserving of attention when perused in the seclusion of the study."
Sir Walter Scott in "Rob Roy"

The previous chapter dealt with the purpose of stories, this one explores how we understand and interpret stories. If it is accepted that stories form a fundamental part of life then the meaning of them has some significance. The range of different types of stories was outlined in the first chapter, and it is clear that each genre will mean different things to different people at different times. Fairy stories, for example, have a particular function with children, to delight, mystify and entrance. To professors of psychology and anthropology they provide deeper meanings and connect as to streams of universal and unconscious thought. Thus there may be no single or common way to understand stories, indeed that would be an anathema. Stories mean what you and I want them to mean. We interpret them ourselves, for ourselves. This chapter considers first the nature and structure of stories and narrative, and draws on the very wide literature in this field. It will then consider how we interpret stories, the importance of listening skills, and looks at medical stories in this context. The particular issue of humourous stories will be covered in subsequent chapters.

The nature and structure of stories. Stories, or narratives, come in many forms. They were, of course, in oral form at the beginning until the use of writing fixed them at a period of time. This distinction between oral and written is crucial. The language changes when the story is written and the written form generally precludes further change and development of the narrative. The context of reading a story and listening to it, is quite different. Taking down a story told by someone loses in some cases the essence of the tale. The analogy with case histories of patients is obvious at this stage. The short summary in the case notes is only that, a summary, and can miss some essential parts of the tale.

In a similar way as we try to understand a story, again consider case histories, the language we use is different from the original. We use technical terms and structure the story in a particular way. The emphasis may be changed and the key features modified.

The role of editors is especially important in this respect. A story is told by an individual, reported on by an observer, and then edited. The headline, the paragraph break-up and the structure can all be modified, and thus change the meaning of the original. Finally, of course, in this introduction, the language used is critical to the meaning of the story. Indeed one of the most interesting parts of story telling is the interpretation of the meaning of individual words in the context of the tale, the exegesis. This term, an important one in the understanding of stories is discussed in more detail later in this chapter.

What are stories? There is a very considerable literature on this subject and the following brief review does no more than point the reader at the richness of the material available (see for example, Hawthorn, 1997. Ong, 1996. Chatman, 1978. Sautman et al, 1998). The following quotations are illustrative only, but give some feeling for the subject. They all come from books relevant to the process of narrative.

McEwan and Egan (1995) make some important points.

"A list is not a narrative... what distinguishes a narrative is that it takes shape...has a rhythm that ultimately springs from patterns important in human life and action."

"A story, deals not just in facts or ideas or theories, or even dreams, but in facts and draws from the perspective of someone's life and in the context of someone's emotions."

Cohan and Shires (1988) define stories as follows.

"A story consists of events placed in a sequence to delineate the process of change, the transformation of one event into another. The events depict some sort of physical or mental activity, an occurrence in the events of a story do not occur in isolation but belong to a sequence."

Todorof (1977) uses the following.

"An ideal narrative begins with a stable situation which is disturbed by some power or force. There results in a state if dis-equilibrium; by the action of a force directed in the opposite direction, the equilibrium is re-established; the second equilibrium is similar to the first, but the two are never identical."

There is thus a sequence which sets out the main elements of the story over time though there can be satellite or additional events which occur. The contrasts, and similarities, to the medical story in this respect are interesting. The patient's story, presented as a history, may be a logical sequence, with all the clues in the right order. But it may not. The medical story is much more like a detective story in which the author alters the sequence, misses out key events, leads the reader down the wrong pathway, until there is a denouement. The key in medical stories is getting the sequence right. Good stories invite you to be part of the process, to be involved in the action and feel part of the solution. For patients this is essential. They are their own story and they need to continue to be part of the continuing process of discussion and management. There are many reasons why patients and the public need to be involved, continuing to be part of their own story journey is just one of them. The doctor also becomes involved and part of the story, changing it, adding to it and in some instances completely re-writing it.

It is well recognised that tests, investigations and clinical procedures used in medical practice are not always infallible and there are both false positives and negatives. It remains important, therefore, that the doctor listens to the patient and should the results of the "tests" not fit the clinical picture, they should be reviewed.

The characters in the story are also important. Authors may spend a considerable time and great skill in sketching in the character. In some books it is the characters, not the plot which are most memorable. The establishment of the character of the leading persons sets the tone for the story, and so it is in clinical practice. It would be difficult to understand and to help manage a complex clinical problem without understanding the patient and ensuring that the patient was part of the process. Patients are the characters at the heart of clinical stories.

Narrative links human actions and emotions and puts then together in a way which makes sense and is cohesive. In this respect stories help us to understand life and its meaning. They could therefore be considered to have an educational purpose, by informing, interpreting and imparting both knowledge and attitudes. In this respect they can be used as recollections, anecdotes, illustrations and examples. Good teachers are those who can construct and structure stories (teaching material) to best effect and thus guide our way through a subject. They act as guides only, the student or learner must then reconstruct the story for him or herself to make it meaningful. They have to be able to tell the story in their own words, hence the relevance of essay writing and oral performance in assessing competence for professional groups. The learning should be deep enough to allow more than rote learning and regurgitation of the facts. It should provide the learner with an opportunity to present the topic in his or her own way. They transform the subject into a form which corresponds with their own concept map. Note taking, within a teaching context or at the bedside is thus an essential part of the process. The summaries which are written present our own views and interpretation of the topic, or the clinical problem presented by the patient. This subject is described in more detail in Chapter 6.

It is possible sometimes, using the same "text", to modify the presentation of the story and indeed use different language. For example, the same story may be narrated differently to medical students, at a postgraduate seminar or at a formal lecture, or to a public group. As the context changes so does the language. This also illustrates the power of the oral presentation. It can be modified, extended, and different analogies and examples used for different audiences. The audience is thus part, an active part, of the presentation. As such they are capable, even in a formal teaching sense, of being modified and changed. This is part of the creative process, and of good teaching. The development within a learning programme of teaching material which stimulates the imagination and which is readily remembered and understood is one of the delights of teaching practice. Think of the stories related through Socrates by Plato. Such stories are still discussed and remembered. Powerful stories always are. The great sagas, tales and books over the generations show just how much impact they have, and continue to have. Re-reading the classics is a wonderful experience (see Annexe 1).

Stories can be classified into different genres, in an arbitrary way. These include epics, romances, comedies, tragedies, thrillers, science fiction, westerns, detective novels and mysteries. The structure of each of these may be different and some may correspond more to the definitions, given previously, than others. As mentioned previously, medical stories are perhaps more like detective stories, but there are obviously elements of mystery, tragedy, comedy and science fiction. Comedy will be discussed in the next chapter

The concept of the doctor as a detective is one which is not well enough recognised. Much of what we do is based on curiosity and a wish to find out what the problem is. We follow clues, and are led up blind alleys just like Poirot or Morse. We test hypotheses and match them to the story and the presenting features. We may even try an intervention, with the patient's full consent, to see if the culprit can be revealed.

It is interesting to note that it is not possible to become involved in and understand a specialised genre (such as the medical story) without some background and to engage in the subject via stories. It is necessary to have some basic concepts and understanding, otherwise the special area loses its impact and meaning. For example the language used is generally different and the concepts need to be fully appreciated before the relevance of the tale can be appreciated. Hence the possibility of keeping outsiders away from the mysteries of the profession or group. This process is of course directly relevant to learning. It is essential that the learner has sufficient background before starting to learn a subject or it will be much more difficult or even meaningless. This topic will be discussed further in Chapter 5.

The interpretation of stories. One of the most interesting aspects of story telling is how we interpret stories and make sense of them. The science behind this is called hermeneutics, and the interpretation of individual stories, or indeed lines or words in stories is exegesis. (Try using the term in a meeting and gauge the reaction.) This latter term is more commonly used in the study of biblical texts where a verse or a word are debated and discussed. A similar process occurs in staff rooms and committees across the country as health care professionals and managers try to interpret the latest Government circular. Journal clubs and seminars provide the same setting for the interpretation of the written word, or the story of a patient. What was meant by that statement? Why was that word used and not another? How can this concept be related to others? In clinical terms this relates to such questions as, what does that symptom mean? Why was this test positive? Why was this intervention not effective? This is the bread and butter of clinical audit, professional review and continuing education. It is part of the role of the doctor and is essential for the development of trust between the patient and the professional.

As a first step it is possible to consider how we interpret patient stories. Every patient is unique in the story that they tell. The chances are, however, that even their special story will fit into a pattern which will suggest a particular illness or diagnosis. In one sense that is the purpose of telling the story, in order to make sense of it and to help with the problem. The skill in doing this is two fold. First, to listen to the story carefully and actively synthesise the key aspects, and coming to a tentative conclusion which will be amplified by examination and investigations if required. This is the core or the kernel of the story. It is the second part which is just as important. It is the understanding of the feelings, emotions, fears such as anger and anxiety which overlie the core. This is the part of the story which will be just as important when discussions on management will be undertaken. It is the part of the story which establishes the character and person behind the disease. Great authors do this wonderfully and doctors have the privilege of doing it on a daily basis.

Complex patient stories can be very difficult to interpret and can take time, skill and patience. In contrast to fictional narrative, patient stories may not have a simple solution and the equilibrium re-established on the final page. There may be no explanation for the illness and the interpretation of such stories can be very difficult. Many of the illnesses faced by general practitioners are not capable of identification. They may be due to "virus" or a "strain" or even "stress", but this does not explain them, only gives them a name. This of course is a common failing of professional groups. Giving a name to a problem does not solve it, though it may make the patient feel that at last a solution has been found. A cartoon caption stated "At last Mr Drabble we've identified your illness. You have Drabbles disease", makes the point clearly. Together the patient and the doctor will need to come to some interpretation of the problem even if it is "don't know". However as the story unfolds the understanding of the problem may become clearer.

The "don't know" answer is also important. Some years back it would have been very difficult for the doctor to say that. It wasn't done and the doctor would lose face. How could he (and it usually was a he) say that he didn't know. Yet in the development of trust patients need to be aware of the uncertainties in medicine and the management of this can be one of the most difficult tasks in medicine. Part of the discussion relates to how we individually perceive a story. Tell a story to a group of people, ask them all to watch a television programme, or present a patient (his)story to them. Ask them to write down what their views are on the story, the main points, the key issues. The chances are that they will emphasise different issues. It is always a salutary exercise to ask students to write down at the end of a lecture the key points that they thought important and compare it to your own. In the clinical setting the same is true, especially if there are different health care professionals present. We all interpret stories in the light of our own experience and background. It is not possible to avoid this. Different professional groups, and even different specialties within medicine, will interpret problems differently and are therefore likely to offer different solutions. It is necessary to understand this, and also to recognise the impact this may have on patient care. With the development of teams and interdisciplinary working this is likely to become even more evident. The recognition that others will see things differently, and may even disagree with each other is certainly possible. Kant said "We see things not as they are, but as we are". We all make our own interpretations of stories, and that makes life richer and fuller. Others can often throw shafts of light on a problem seen from a different perspective, and this should be encouraged for the benefit of patients.

The psychological component of the story has always attracted particular attention in relation to interpretation. Psychoanalysis is based on this aspect of listening and in itself it is therapeutic. But this should be part of the whole process of listening and interpreting. The meaning of words, phrases, symbols and dreams are all relevant. The non-verbal part of the story, gestures, expressions and eye contact all add to the story and cannot be easily encaptured in a few phrases in the case notes. They are essential for the second part of the interpretation process, that of explaining the problem and helping with its solution.

Above all, listening to the patient is the most important part of the process. Time is always a factor. We never have enough. But the story is perhaps the most relevant part of the process of making a diagnosis and in setting out a course of action with the patient.

Listening skills. It should be obvious from the discussion that listening forms a key part of storytelling, and that the listener has to be seen to listen. There can be fewer more frustrating issues than having explained something in great detail, to hear the response, "What did you say?" This is part of everyday life, but if you are unwell, angry and frightened you need someone to listen to you. Some tales are of course enthralling, and it is impossible not to feel involved. However at the end of a busy clinic it is more difficult to replicate the freshness at its beginning. There are skills to be developed in active and creative listening. This is more than just nodding the head at irregular intervals, it involves giving time and space to another person. There are times during the process when interventions, questions, are helpful. There are other occasions when the individual needs to speak, uninterrupted. Training in this area has progressed enormously over the years, and is now seen to be part of "communication skills" courses. Watching a good listener is part of this. As a medical student in the early 1960s the author was brought up on a small book on "Clinical Methods." Here is how communication is described.

"**The interrogation of the patient.** The object of interrogation is to elicit information regarding the patient's present illness, the state of his previous health and that of his family. The interrogation must be patiently carried out, the patient being allowed, as far as possible, to tell his story in his own words. One patient is a good witness and another poor. One gives an excellent history. Another has to have the history of his illness dragged out of him by methods of slow extortion, and even then a great deal of what he says may prove irrelevant. Some patients seem quite unable to give any precise account of what they feel to be wrong. This may be due to stupidity or the effects of disease on their mental faculties."

So much for instilling confidence and trust! Fortunately, those who taught the author of this book made up for the shortcomings illustrated above by their compassion and example. They were heroes.

In a course on literature and medicine at the University of Glasgow (Calman et al 1988) the class studied "The Cocktail Party" by T.S. Eliot. The first act of the play is set at a cocktail party with the guests talking but not listening to each other. It was a fourth year student who said "but that's what we do to patients". In saying this she showed great maturity and an understanding of the process of listening.

Dealing with uncertainty. As has already been discussed in this chapter medical stories sometimes do not have a neat or perfect ending. Most other types of story do, even complicated and challenging detective novels. This means that the problem of uncertainty remains and it may not be possible to know the end of the story or sometimes even its direction of travel. The never-ending story can be a real phenomenon in medical practice. This means that explaining the patient journey can be very difficult as it changes and is altered by the progression of the disease and the effects of treatment. It is a time when trust between the patient and the doctor needs to be real and effective. Trust is at the heart of the relationship and no apology is made for repeating this at regular intervals.

The transformational impact of stories. Stories can change people and the course of events. They can have an enormously powerful effect on behaviour. While this will be discussed in more detail in chapter 9, under the title "The contagious theory of behaviour change" it is raised at this point as we try to understand stories and their impact. Parables and fables have already been mentioned as ways in which the telling of a tale can illustrate "good" and "bad". They can also be used in educational settings and as examples. Thus a story about the way in which a particular patient was dealt with can lead to questions about the therapy and the science as well as the communication of information and the behaviour of the staff. The student or junior doctor can thus ask questions about him or her self, and whether or not they would react in the same way. Negative behaviour, if reinforced at the clinical level can also act to change the way in which a new doctor acts. As has been said previously the hidden curriculum is very powerful in medicine. Teachers plan the stories they use with great care to explain and to amplify the factual base of the curriculum.

Stories also come as part of the knowledge base, and it would be impossible to think about stories without considering this. They are more than just tales which excite and amuse. The also provide a diet of facts and evidence. We learn from stories and use then to transmit knowledge and information. They supplement the other ways of learning.

Creating a new story. One of the most exciting things to do in medicine is to write, or create, a new story, one which has never been told before. This requires originality, imagination, and an ability to think beyond what is currently happening and being prepared to create something different. It can be done in any setting; the laboratory, the clinic, the operating theatre, the community or in front of a computer. It will require curiosity and a desire to do things better, and to open new ways of thinking.

There is an aboriginal proverb which says "there are no paths, paths are made by walking". One of the roles of the doctor is to make new paths and to go where no woman or man has gone before. The words of Robert Frost ring true for those who have written new tales.

> "I shall be telling this with a sigh
> Somewhere ages and ages hence
> Two roads diverged in a wood. And I
> Took the road less travelled by
> And that has made all the difference."

We need people in medicine who are able to change things and not to be frightened to take a different path.

Some special aspects of medical stories. One of the most interesting aspects of medical stories is the language in which they are written. They use abbreviations and unusual words which can only be understood by those who have been initiated. These are intimidating and infuriating. Doctors are of course no different from any other professional group, but this is no excuse. We talk over and through patients. We stand above them and discuss their bodies and feelings across them as if they were not there. Thus, not only the language but the context matters. Sit in an outpatient clinic and watch what happens. The powerful institutional setting diminishes the patient and the language used makes it difficult for them to take part in the process. There is a superiority (not only by doctors, but the whole team) which can inhibit the development of the relationship between professional and patient. The context also dictates who can speak, and when, and how much control one has over the process.

SOME CONCLUSIONS

This chapter set out to try to explain why stories are important and to understand their function. It is clear that there are many different types of story, but that medical stories fit the pattern well in general respects. However, they are different in the language they use and in the context within which they are told. The interpretation of stories is a key role of the doctor, and it is particularly difficult when there is uncertainty. Writing a new story is a very special part of being a doctor.

REFERENCES.

Calman, K.C, Downie, R.S, Duthie, M, and Sweeney,B. Literature and medicine: A course. 1988, Medical Education, 22, 265-69.

Chatman, S. Story and Discourse. Narrative structure in fiction and film. 1978. Cornell University Press.

Cohan, S. and Shires, L.M. Telling Stories. A theoretical analysis of narrative fiction. 1988, Routledge, London and New York.

Hawthorn, J. Studying the Novel. An introduction. 1997, Third Edition. Arnold, London.

McEwan, H and Egan,K. Narrative in Teaching, Learning and Research. 1995. Teachers College Press, Columbia University, New York.

Ong, W.J. Orality and Literacy. The technologising of the world. 1982, (1996 reprint) Routledge, London and New York.

Sautman, F.C, Conchado, D, and Di Scipio, G.C. Telling Tales. Medieval narratives and the folk tradition, 1998. Macmillan Press, Basingstoke.

Todorof, T. The Politics of Prose. 1977, Ithica, New York, Cornell University Press.

4. Humour

"One deterrent to the study of humour, is that as soon as one starts examining humour, or dissecting jokes, it loses its appeal, spontaneity and directness, and may appear trivial. Analysing a joke has been compared to dissecting a frog. Once the dissection has been completed, we are more informed about the anatomy, but the frog is dead." *Haig, in "The Anatomy of Humour."*

Introduction. Humour is a serious matter, and even a publication such as The Economist (remember Carlisle's phrase about economics as the "dismal science") has written about it (The Economist, December 1997, p25-27). The jokes they use to illustrate the article at least made someone laugh. The introductory heading to the piece, "To understand a country, you can study its economic data or demographic statistics. Or you can collect its jokes." There are of course many ways in which humour can be delivered, and one of these is through stories. Humourous stories. But why do we laugh and smile at such stories, and is there a purpose behind it? Is there any benefit in humour and laughter?

This chapter sets out to look at four aspects of humour. The first is the mechanism of laughter and the anatomy and physiology behind it. The second is to consider a series of writings on humour. The purpose of this being to try to understand what makes us laugh. The third is to bring together some thoughts on why we need to laugh as well as some of the benefits that may bring. Finally there will be a discussion on medical humour. It should be noted at this stage that humans are the only animals who laugh, which raises issues of the possible evolutionary benefits of laughter.

The physiology of laughter. Laughter is a subject which is surprisingly well understood. Herbert Spenser in a classic essay "On the physiology of laughter" written in 1860, details out some of the muscle groups involved and comments on its purpose. Darwin also wrote on the subject "On the Expression of Emotion in Men and Animals" in 1872 and he devotes a whole chapter to "Joy, high spirits and love." Again he lists the muscle groups involved and quotes the work of Duchenne (1862), on muscle movement. He uses a wonderful phrase to describe laughter, and says that it is "the tickling of the mind". He also makes a most interesting comment on music in the same section of the book, a topic which will be developed further in this volume.

"Music has a wonderful power, as I have attempted elsewhere to show, of recalling in a vague and indefinite manner, those strong emotions which were felt during long-past ages, when, as is probable, our early progenitors courted each other by the aid of vocal tones. And as several of our strongest emotions - grief, great joy, love, and sympathy - lead to the free secretions of tears, it is not surprising that music should be apt to cause our eyes to become suffused with tears."

More recent writing, for example by Hauser et al (Laughter Down the Centuries, 1997) describes the range of muscle groups which are involved, much of which is based on the studies of Duchenne (1862) who stimulated individual muscles and observed the effect. This has been further developed by Williams et al (1989) in Gray's Anatomy 37th Edition. The muscle groups include zygomaticus major and minor, levator anguli oris muscle, levator labii superioris, part of the levator labii superioris alaeque nasi and the risorius muscle. They act in combination and the patterns of activity which can result range from a smile to full laughter. They are also associated with forced expiratory sounds. We can even hurt ourselves laughing as we "split our sides".

Laughter begins at around four months of age and is proceeded by smiling. It can be elicited by touch and noise and by tickling. Certain parts of the body are particularly associated with tickling such as the sole of the foot, the axilla, the ribs and the abdomen. Darwin (1872) linked this, as has been already alluded to as the "tickling of the mind" and looked at the relationship between laughter from tickling and that associated with a humourous story or event. One being categorised as a reflex action the other associated with similar brain activity (Fridlund and Loftis, 1990).

There is thus much muscular movement in laughing and this may account for some of its potential benefits. It is triggered by many things and in the adult it is usually because of some activity or sensation which is seen to be funny. What exactly is "funny" is of course a matter of opinion, and varies from person to person. Some of us seem to laugh more readily than others. This takes us to the second section in which the possibility of explaining humour is considered.

Some writings on humour. Over the centuries much has been written about humour and the theories behind it. This is similar to humourous writing, which is also of great antiquity. It could be argued that trying to analyse humour, as the introductory quotation to this chapter states, is inappropriate, that it will destroy laughter and happiness in an attempt to rationalise it and categorise it. This is a legitimate point of view which is however rejected for the following reasons. First, it is important to understand biological phenomena, and humour and laughter is certainly one of these. Why should we not try to understand something which is important to all of us, and which is peculiarly human? Second, if humour has a biological function (such as the improvement of well being) then the mechanism by which this operates might give insights into how health and quality of life can be improved. If there is a molecular or physiological mechanism we should try to find out what it is. Third, it is possible that humour is related to other important functions such as learning and creativity, and indeed this is assumed in the thrust of this book. If this is the case then any insights into such an area would be valuable. Finally wouldn't it be nice to know how to make people laugh and enjoy themselves. It is an essential part of wellbeing, and happiness is something to be wished for. It is part of the health and the quality of life of all of us.

The following section is in no sense exhaustive but is an attempt at giving a flavour of the kind of literature available, which is extensive.

Aristotle. In the "Ethics", Aristotle tackles the question of humour and wit. He sees humour and comedy as legitimate aspects of happiness and relaxation, but not as important as seriousness. Happiness, he says, must be distinguished from amusement. Relaxation is not seen as an end in itself and a happy life is to be lived in accordance with goodness, and this is serious and does not consist in amusing oneself. He relates humour and wit to conversations and distinguishes between wit and buffoonery. He makes the point that the boor is useless at social intercourse, contributes nothing, and takes offence at every thing. Those who exercise their humour with good taste are called witty. Relaxation and amusement are essential to living a full life.

Plato. Many of the Socratic dialogues contain humourous passages but the classic comment is in the "Philebus" (paras 48ff) where comedy is seen to be part of pain and pleasure. Even in tragedy while the audience is weeping they are enjoying themselves. He uses the concept of "spite" to illustrate that a spiteful person is pleased at his neighbour's misfortunes. Not just on the stage but in real life comedy and tragedy are mixed. From this we might conclude that humourous situations may have their dark side and that pleasure for one person, especially if the situation relates to a misfortune or to an accident, might be pain to another. The classic is the slipping on a banana skin, a funny moment, unless real injury is caused when the pain affects both the observer and the person who slips.

Joubert. Joubert was a medieval physician who wrote a treatise on laughter in 1560. He believed like Plato that joy and sadness are experienced by the heart and not the mind. Sadness caused the heart to retract, while happiness caused dilatation. As the heart was tethered to the diaphragm by the pericardium, so the alternating contractions moved the diaphragm and caused laughter. He also noted that excessive laughter might be harmful and could cause digestive upsets, coughing and occasionally death. (Joubert, L A Treatise on Laughter. 1980, University of Alabama Press.)

Robert Burton. Burton's book, "The Anatomy of Melancholy" written in the early 17th century, is a quite remarkable work, covering a huge range of topics all more or less related to melancholy and its correction. He too refers to the power of musick as a remedy for melancholy to "exhilarate a sorrowful heart". But his reference to the value of mirth is even more effusive.

"Mirth purgeth the blood, confirms health, causes a fresh pleasing, and fine colour, prorogues life, whets the wit, makes the body young, lively and fit for any manner of employment. The merrier the heart the longer the life."

He goes on to describe the conditions required, including good company, song, wine and merryment. In a subsequent chapter on "Medicines" and their power to make people happy he relates their value and their disadvantages and discusses the medicines that apothecaries mix in their shops. Overall he does not see any real benefit from medication and indeed he says, "Many cavil at this type of physick, and hold it unnecessary, unprofitable to this or any other disease, because those countries which use it least live longest, and are best in health, as Hector

Boethius relates of the Isles of Orcades, the people are still sound of body and mind without any use of physick, and they commonly live 120 years."

William Hazlitt. In his "Lectures on English Comic Writers" written in 1818, Hazlitt makes the well-known point that man is the only animal who laughs and weeps. Wit he says "is the salt of conversation, not the food". There is thus a danger of overdoing humour. It is not possible to force people to laugh, and conversely even formal occasions can be funny if mistakes and misunderstandings take place. Using wit is partly about the pursuit of pleasure. The distinction between wit and humour is worth quoting.

"Humour is the describing of the ludicrous as it is in itself; wit is exposing it by comparing or contrasting it with something else. Humour is the growth of nature and accident. Wit is the product of art and fancy."

Herbert Spenser. Reference has already been made to Spencer's essay on laughter. In it, in addition to describing laughter, he also touches on the functions of laughter. These he lists as defensive, social communication, and aggression. He also notes that you can laugh on your own, without anyone else, but of course one cannot share a joke without others being present.

Henri Bergson. His book on "Laughter" published in English translation in 1913 is one of the most frequently quoted texts on this subject. He emphasises as others do the human nature of laughter. He analyses the situations which result in laughter and relates much of it to physical factors such as deformities and comic expressions. He then considers the role of gestures and movements and links these to the concept of the body as a machine. The use of differences in dress, skin colour and eccentricities are all things that might be laughable. It is the disturbing of the mechanical and the routine which can result in a humourous situation. It is the unusual, the absurd and the strange which are funny. The contrast between the normal and the abnormal and the sudden change from the expected to the unexpected. The punch-line of the joke make the same point as the twist in the tale, or the denouement of the story. Ridicule and making fun of people he sees as part of this picking on weaknesses and rigid regulations. He quotes Doctor Bahis in Molière's "L'amour Médecin" "It is better to die through following the rules than to recover through violating them." The mechanical and routine being ridiculed, and made fun of.

Sigmund Freud. In 1905 Freud published "De witz und seine Beziehung zum Ubewussten" whose English translation "Jokes and their relation to the unconscious" was first published in 1916. It is a remarkable book, full of Jewish jokes and their analysis. To the reader who thinks of Freud as one of the most serious and influential figures of the 20th century the book will come as something of a surprise. Yet it should not be so. The history of the analysis of humour, noted above, links pleasure to pain, sees amusement in the faults of others, which may be one of the driving forces in seeking happiness.

He considers the technique of jokes, some of which abbreviate, are a play on words, use puns, or are silly jokes. He considers the purpose of jokes which may be innocent or hostile. This latter comes up regularly in the literature, jokes and humour have a black side. Humour also allows us to consider taboo subjects and as Freud comments this ensures that jokes "Evade restrictions and open sources of pleasure that have become inaccessible". Jokes can be for play, but they may also be for power, and can be used to dominate and "put down". He also notes that more than one person is required if the joke is to be enjoyed, and that they all need to understand and be part of the group before it is funny. "Every joke calls for a public of its own and laughing at the same jokes is evidence of far reaching psychical conformity."

His other comments relate to jokes as "work" and he links this to "dreamworks". "For the euphoria which we endeavour to reach by these means is nothing other than the mood of a period of life in which we were accustomed to deal with our psychic work in general with a small expenditure of energy - the mood of our childhood, when we were ignorant of the comic, when we were incapable of jokes and when we had no need for humour to make us feel happy in our life." The significance of "work" in this process will be developed further in a subsequent chapter.

It is not therefore surprising that a psychoanalytic approach, looking for motivating factors, and unconscious drivers, has be carried out. This fascinating book covers a very wide range of issues, the jokes are splendid and it is worth a read.

Arthur Koestler. His book, "The Act of Creation" was one of the starting points for this current book. It is a splendid analysis of the links between learning, humour and the ability to create new ideas. The thesis is that they are connected by the way in which different ideas come together in sparking off new thoughts. It is the "Eureka" response in which there are sudden insights into a problem. He links humour with discovery and learning and with problem solving. Creating humour is like the process of scientific discovery. In humour, Koestler would argue the joke is "seen" when two different ideas are brought together in a distinctive way. That is when we laugh or smile. This fits into more recent thinking on the concept of "epiphany", a recognition of something new and different appearing.

He quotes Greig from "The Psychology of Laughter and Comedy" (1923) as saying, "Humour is the only domain where a stimulus on a high level of complexity produces a massive and sharply defined response on the level of physiological reflexes". It is thus a very sophisticated response which results in a reflex which has origins in our past. He also quotes from Hobbes in the "Leviathan" who says "The passion of laughter is nothing else but a sudden glory arising from a sudden conception of some emenancy in ourselves by comparison with the infirmity of others, or with our own formerly." We do laugh at others, and at ourselves.

He also makes a fascinating reference to the infectious nature of laughter and humour which is directly relevant to the Transmid theory. "The bacillus of laughter is a bug difficult to isolate: once brought under the microscope it will turn out to be a yeast-like universal ferment equally useful in making wine or vinegar or bread."

This book is one which must be read if one has an interest in humour, learning and creativity. It is full of insights, stories and examples.

Stephen Potter.   Potter writing in the 1950s reviews English humour in his book "The Sense of Humour", and tries to define it. He then uses numerous examples to illustrate the point. Such anthologies and collections of prose, comic poetry or jokes are readily come by, but few try to analyse the background. Potter reviews the literature on the subject and concludes that humour is about the release of inhibitions and he, in a rather negative way, discusses the irrelevance of laughter. Perhaps it has no point. Finally in his conclusions he quotes Coleridge who noted that the first excellence of Sterne was the "bringing forward into distinct consciousness those minutiae of thought and feeling which appear trifles, have an importance only for the moment, and yet almost every man feels in one way or another". He makes the point that humour at its highest can be near to poetry. Perhaps most originally he connects this to the "sense" of humour. A feeling of consciousness, and as Freud might say of unconsciousness, like our other senses able to be stimulated and in doing so add a new dimension to like. Like sight, touch and hearing an indispensable "sense" for everyone.

Robin Haig **(1988)** wrote a very full review of the subject with a book entitled "The Anatomy of Humour" (Charles C Thomas, Springfield Illinois.) As well as being an excellent summary of the literature he also introduces a new theory, that of Gelastic Gain,(Gelastic: serving the function of humour.) He defines this theory as follows, "Laughter, a biological phenomenon in homo sapiens, occurs spontaneously when there is a sudden perception by the subject of a net gain in emotional cognitive, social or material assets, and functions as a social signal to communicate this gain". He goes on to say that the theory is derived from the fact that object loss is associated with distress and crying. He has a fascinating table contrasting grief and good humour. He notes in particular that the cognitive processing of jokes is often very rapid (within seconds). There is a real gain in being happy and it gives a sense of security. He records that Lorenz (1963) also claimed that the social origin of laughter arose from the signalling of security to other members of the group (Lorenz, K, On Aggression. New York, Harcourt, Brace, 1963.) Perhaps this is another component of the evolutionary benefits of laughter.

Some interim conclusions. So what do all these studies, and there are many more, add up to. For the most part they are descriptions of humour and its characteristics rather than a detailed analysis of the mechanisms. We can describe the physiology of laughing, but cannot explain the mechanism which triggers it. Nor can we describe, other than in a most general way what makes one thing funny and another not. Clearly some event, external or internal, sets off a whole series of actions which results in laughter. The external events are very varied, and range from jokes to situations, from visual images to sound, from literature to mime, the list is endless. The internal triggers are also of some interest. It is possible for us to think in a humourous way. We can dream up and create amusing events and situations. We can compose, write, perform and entertain for the benefit of others. So some people know how to do it, and do it rather well. Comedians, using their own material, or pieces written by others give us hours of pleasure. They must have a feeling for what will make people laugh and they generally get it right, though those who have performed at the old Glasgow Empire will recognise that this may not be universally the case. Humour also seems to have an evolutionary function in that it gives us some security of existence and gives us reasoning and control over nature.

But what can the neurophysiological mechanism be? It must generally be in response to some stimulus as perceived by one or more of the senses. This must then be converted into a nervous or endocrine response which results in laughing, and the muscular contractions which are visibly seen and expressed. Is there a laughter centre which when stimulated responds? How are degrees of response controlled? In other words why do we sometimes just smile and at other times cry with laughter? Is there a genetic predisposition to being "funny" or to being someone who has a "sense of humour?" Will the human genome project be able to identify the laughter gene?

In a later section of this book the "Contagious Theory of Behaviour Change" will be outlined. In brief it states that ideas and values are transmitted from one person to another, via the senses, by Transmids. Humour, it is considered, in the same way. Laughter is communicated from person to person, and it changes their perception of the subject. It certainly has a gain, and it has a social function. Freud's concern with "work" in the mind may be of a similar nature.

These may seem to be rather silly questions, and perhaps they are. However if one of the functions of medicine is to improve well being and quality of life then answers to them, or similar questions, matters to you and me and to our patients. There is a huge clinical problem in the clinical setting of depression and anxiety and "stress". We spend millions of pounds on drug therapy and in consultations. If, as we shall examine in the next section, there is some therapeutic benefit from laughter, then it could become a legitimate subject for research. The Medical Research Council and the Wellcome Trust might even consider a pro-active research programme to cover this. And, as was suggested in the preface, there might even be a change in name in Whitehall to the Department of Health and Happiness.

The next section of this chapter tries to answer the question, is there a therapeutic benefit from laughter, humour and being happy?; but first a collection of quotations about the link between laughter and health. They show how deeply the two are related in our culture.

> "Humour is the best medicine." *Anon.*
> "Laughter is the best medicine" *Robert Burton.*
> "The best doctors in the world are Doctor Diet, Doctor Quiet, and Doctor Merryman." *Jonathan Swift.*
> "The first end of comedy is delight, and instruction only the second." *Dryden*
> "Being cheerful keeps you healthy." *Proverbs.*
> "The best of healers is good cheer" *Pindar*

It should perhaps be noted that the Bible has 29 references to laughter, 27 of these refer to scorn and derision and only 2 to joy and happiness.

The benefits of laughter, is laughter therapeutic? Intuitively it seems right. When you read a book, watch a film or a video, listen to the radio, which contains something amusing, you feel better. You may even want to tell someone about it, and it puts you in a good mood. But what is the evidence that it does really make a difference? Is there any objective evidence to support the intuition?

In 1872 Darwin recognised that laughter was specific to man and was part of our inheritance. It is universal and, in general, the same expressions are recognised across all cultures. The relationship between laughter and crying is complex but one can lead to the other. It is possible to laugh or cry with joy. The work of Berk (cited in Zeigler, J. 1995) indicates that people may be helping themselves by laughing. It causes the nostrils to flair, the diaphram and abdominal muscles to contract. Heart rate and blood pressure increase and there is some vasodilation. It is followed by a period of relaxation. A good laugh stimulates a number of muscle groups and improves the circulation. There are also effects on the brain and there is enhancement of the production of endorphins, and the immune system may respond more appropriately to disease (Zeigler, 1995).

In this respect it is possible to conclude that laughter stimulates a number of physiological changes which are generally beneficial. It seems physically good for us, and laughing on a regular basis keeps the blood flowing, the immune system primed, and the muscles pumping. Just as importantly the relaxation afterwards has a positive benefit. For those who are "stressed" and unable to relax, then perhaps this is one way to help. However as will be clear in subsequent sections of this chapter, more research is needed.

There are a number of studies looking at the impact on health. These include, Cousins, 1989, Schmidtt, 1990, Davidhizar and Bowen, 1992, Erdman, 1991, Pasquali, 1990, Tennant, 1990. In cancer patients, the elderly, in stress situations and those with psychosocial problems the benefits seem to be real. It helps with well being and self esteem. The evolutionary benefit may therefore be in the ability to deal with stress more effectively, as a tension relieving mechanism and as a way of relaxing and at the same time activating a number of important physiological mechanisms, which improve circulation and respiration. The release and relief of laughter and humour are clear. They help us cope more effectively.

There are also some other benefits. These include the improvement of communication, and the ability to make a particular point with great effectiveness. Laughter and humour are also very creative experiences and they can be useful in learning about a subject. As Koestler has pointed out the relationship between humour, creativity and learning is a strong one.

A particular aspect of humour is the need both to understand the context, and have sufficient knowledge to follow the humour. It is in this way that it is similar to learning. A sufficient level of knowledge is necessary otherwise the point of the joke is lost. Thus "in jokes" can only be understood in a particular context and are often dated if the context is lost. Part of being a professional, and a specialist, is that the jokes and the humour are so selective that only those in "the circle" can understand. It is for this reason that the writer of this book has suggested that professional exams should also contain jokes. If the candidate does not laugh then they cannot properly be admitted to the professional group.

The health benefits are thus beginning to be documented but clearly more work still needs to be done. The publicity surrounding the work of Patch Adams in his book (Gesundheit, 1998) and the recent film, may stimulate more work, though the funding bodies may still wish to take a cautious view. The Adams book also contains numerous references to the publications on humour and healing.

A recent literature search under the heading "Therapeutic aspects of humour" revealed over 80 references over the past 10 years. Many of these are discursive and anecdotal, and add little to our understanding of the value of humour. However, some are of considerable interest. For example, the role of humour in group psychotherapy has been described, but it notes also the potential destructive nature of humour (Bloch, Browning and Mcgrath,1983). Its role in depression and suicidal patients has also been described and there was symptom relief and reduction of stress (Richman, 1995). More interesting perhaps is the value of humour in the raising of the pain threshold. Two publications, (Weisenberg et al, 1995 and Cogan et al, 1987) both describe experimental situations in which subjects were randomised to humour (film or tape) and then the pain threshold tested. In both cases the pain threshold was increased after humour. However a group which watched a "repulsive" film also increased the threshold. The possibility remains however that humour may be of significant clinical benefit.

It was reported in The Times (9.4.00) that an Italian surgeon uses film to calm patients down while they undergo surgery under local anaesthesia. Different films are used for different audiences. Men liking swashbuckling films, and women softer ones. The surgery was seen to be less traumatic. He is quoted that the only drawback is that the operations finished before the films and the patients had then to buy the video to see the ending.

Humour in Medicine. Medical humour is a subset of humour in general, and even the revered journal the Lancet had an editorial on the subject (Lancet, Leading Article, 1998, 351, 1). The subject concerns doctors, illness, medical practice, hospitals and clinics, health and lifestyles. While the characteristics of the humour are the same as other subjects, and the techniques of jokes and situations similar, it is the content and the context which differ. Allusions to bodily functions, anatomical abnormalities, physiological and psychological changes are all part of this. The humour can be "dark" in that it may deal with taboo subjects such as serious illness or death, and with such matters as sexual problems, and surgical operations. It can deal with both success and failure in clinical practice.

The humour is often very specific to individual specialties, and psychiatry, obstetric and urological jokes are common. These "in-jokes" have already been referred to as ways of defining specific groups. This occurs par excellence in medicine. The jokes used to poke fun at each other are generally beneficial.

Different groups tell jokes about other groups. For example, the definition of shifting dullness (which describes the presence or absence of fluid in the abdomen) is often referred to as a "physician's ward round", by surgeons of course. General jokes which take doctors down a peg or too, are also very common, thus,

"Never trust a doctor whose house-plants die."

Individual specialty jokes are very common. Take psychiatrists, and the lightbulb joke.

Q. "How many psychiatrists does it take to change a lightbulb?"
A. "One. But the lightbulb really has to want to change."

And Urologists,

"A patient had been attending a urologist for some time with a bladder problem. One day, it became particularly acute, and he telephoned the hospital. In an attempt to be helpful the receptionist asked where he was ringing from. He replied, "From the waist down"."

But this is not a joke book, and they never seem quite the same written down. For each new development in treatment or diagnosis new jokes are found, whether it is in relation to HIV infection or Viagra. There are many readily available medical joke books, of varying quality, which can be consulted, though they never seem to be quite as funny as they should and don't ever seem so funny as hearing them from someone else. As always the delivery of the joke, the setting of its telling and the timing of the punchline are all important.

There are also some very humourous books about doctors. The "Doctor" stories by Richard Gordon have already been referred to, but there are many others. Of particular interest is Moliere who wrote several plays which included doctors and which are remarkably funny (see Calder, 1993) Moliere's doctors illustrate stupidity, insensitivity, arrogance and ignorance, and taken in good part, that can't be bad. They are obsessed with rights and privileges. In "La malade imaginaire" for example M. Diafoirus says about his son,

"What pleases me most about him, and in this he is following my example, is that he holds blindly to the opinions of our ancients, and he has never wished to understand or listen to the so-called discoveries of our century on the circulation of the blood, and other questions of the same kind."

Re-validation here we come! Calder makes an important general point about humour and Molière. "We are invited, when watching or reading a Molière comedy, to let our understanding be guided by laughter. Every time we laugh or smile, we are making a judgement, and our enjoyment espouses the inner movement of the play and its underlying dialectic. Our pleasure, understanding and moral responses, are indissolubly linked."

Films and television programmes about doctors also have a large contribution to make in amusing and entertaining. The "Carry On" films would be a good example of this, and from the United States, "MASH". This latter had some very serious aspects as well as being extremely funny. The more recent film "Patch Adams", portrays the real story of an American doctor who uses humour regularly in practice and illustrates the potential.

One of the beneficial aspects of humour is in helping staff to cope with difficult situations and crises. It allows difficult problems to be shared and discussed. It is supportive and helps in "team-building" and the development of shared culture and values. The regular use of Christmas shows and reviews in which no individual or group is sacrosanct can only help to open up the organisation and assist in encouraging people to work together.

Increasingly doctors are involved in meetings and working groups. These can take up time and energy, and are sometimes less productive than they should be. In a recent book Kushner (1990) "The Light Touch: How to use humour for business success" the author sets out the many ways in which humour can add to a meeting of management situation. Jokes can be used, he says, in resolving conflict, increasing motivation, assisting in awkward and embarrassing situations, and in improving productivity. He also suggests that this methodology can be used in the writing of memos and letters. Personal experience by the present author suggests that this is indeed the case, though as has been noted in relation to group therapy (a nice way of describing a meeting) it can be destructive and must be used with care and selectively.

Jokes and humour are of interest to teachers as a way of assisting learning. This can be done in a variety of ways from jokes through cartoons or videos. They are often memorable and can help to ensure understanding of a particular point. They can also help the public, in a perverse sort of way, to understand what doctors and other health professionals do. The television programmes which show difficult clinical problems, and make fun of them, can help to transmit knowledge and information. The classic Tony Hancock show, "The Blood Donor" is still talked about, and showed very clearly some of the misconceptions of the process. The public are a very sophisticated group, they understand the issues well, and while further information provision will always be helpful, it is their fears and anxieties which need to be identified, listened to and answered. Humour can help in the process. It can help in the demystification of medicine, and make doctors more accessible and human.

Haig, in his book on "The Anatomy of Humour" has a whole chapter on "Humour, persuasion and education" in which the possible benefits are described. There may be a problem in that humour may divert attention from the subject and may even confuse. D. Zillman and J. Bryant (1983, Uses and Effects of Humour in Educational Ventures. In The Handbook of Humour Research Vol II Eds McGhee,P.E. and Goldstein, J.H , New York, Springer Verlag, pp173-193) note however that there may be some benefit, particularly in children.

An ethical problem? There are a number of ethical issues which need to be raised in relation to the use of humour, one of which is the potential problem of laughing at patients. Is this acceptable? Should we be concerned at the way in which this is done, and does it raise moral issues? Humour can often be cruel and hurtful, and this may even be one of its purposes. Done in the right spirit, then patients may be the subject of jokes and entertainment. However, we always need to be mindful of the potential harm and hurt it may cause. A second problem, already alluded to in an earlier section is that of the role of humour in the dominance of others. In any team setting, such as a clinical unit, it is not difficult to mock or ridicule one or more members of the group. This can be just as cruel as overt bullying.

Humour if it is to be used must be appropriate. Getting it wrong with patients, or indeed one's colleagues can be very disturbing. It can send the wrong signals, alter relationships and inhibit discussion. Humour must therefore be used sparingly in some circumstances, and it is not a cure all, nor a panacea.

SOME CONCLUSIONS

This chapter set out to examine four aspects of humour. The first was to describe the physiology of laughter, and we have seen how the various muscle groups act to produce the outcome. What triggers the laughing response is still unknown, but several hypotheses were presented. The second aspect was to consider a range of writings on humour to see if it could be explained and understood. Various theories have been presented, each with some validity. However, more work does need to be done.

In some ways it is the third section which is of greatest interest, that of the possible benefits of humour. Evidence was presented to show that it does have value in improving well being, improving physiological and psychological functions, and even altering pain thresholds. We feel better and relax more easily. The benefits are therefore real and may be cheaper than the pharmacological alternatives. If this were so then investment in research and development in this area might be worthwhile. Oh to have the first MRC grant on laughter therapy!

Finally the specific aspects of medical humour were discussed. While using the same techniques as other forms of humour the content and context are different. Laughter is important in the medical context for many reasons including teaching and learning, team building, and in increasing the understanding of medical issues in both the profession and the public.

Laughter and having fun are worthwhile and have value for all of us.

REFERENCES

Adams, P and Mylander, M. Gesunheit. 1998, Healing Arts Press Rochester, Vermont.

Bloch,S Browning,S and McGrath, G. Humour in psychotherapy. 1983, Brit J Med. Psychol. 56, 89-97.

Calder,A. Moliere: The Theory and Practice of Comedy. 1993, The Athlone Press, London and the Atlantic Highlands.

Cogan,R., Cogan,D. Waltz, and McCue, 1987, M. Effects of laughter and relaxation on discomfort thresholds,J. Behav. Med. 10, 139-44

Cousins.N ,Anatomy of an Illness as Perceived by the Patient. Reflections on healing and regeneration. Norton, New York1989

Davidhizar,R and Bowen,M. The dynamics of laughter. 1992 Arch Psych Nurs6,132-137.

Duchenne, B. Mecanismede la physiognomie humaine ou analyse electophysiologique de L'expressiondes passions. Bailliere, Paris.

Erdman,L Laughter therapy with patients with cancer. 1991 Oncol. Nurs. Forum.18,1359-63.

Fridlund, A,J and Loftus,J.M Relations between tickling and humourous laughter . 1997 Biological Psychology, 30, 141-150.

Haig, R.A. The Anatomy of Humour. 1988. Charles C. Thomas, Springfield Illinois.

Hauser, G, Rothganger,H., Capellini, A.C. Guidotti, Vienna,A. The Biology of Laughter. Medical, Functional and Anthropological-Human Ethological Aspects. In Laughter Down the Centuries 1997 Turun Yliopisto.

Koestler, A. The Act of Creation. 1964. Hutchison and Co London.

Kushner, M. The Light Touch: How to use humour for business success. 1990, Simon and Schuster, New York.

Pasquali, E.A. Learning to laugh. Humour as therapy. 1990. J Ppsycho Soc Nurs. Ment Health Serv. 28, 31-35.

Richman,J. The lifesaving function of humour with the depressed and suicidal elderly. 1995, Gerontologist, 35, 271-3.

Schmidtt,N. Patients' perception of laughter in a rehabilitation hospital, 1990 Rehabil. Nurs. 15, 143-6.

Tennant, K.F. The effect of humour on the well being of the older adult. 1990 J Gerontol. Nurs.16, 11-17.

Weisenberg,M Tepper,I, and Schwarzwald, Humour as a cognitive technique for increasing pain tolerance. 1995, Pain, 63, 207-12.

Williams,P.L. Warwick,R., Dyson,M., and Bannister L.H. Eds Gray's Anatomy 37th Edition,1989 Churchill Livingstone New York.

Zeigler, J, Immune system may benefit from the ability to laugh. 1995, J. Natl. Cancer Inst. 87, 342-43.

5. Storytelling and Learning

"The basic attraction of medicine for the young student is the opportunity it offers of serving humanity in any one of many ways, for example by helping the sick and infirm, in advancing medical science by research, or by improving the organisation of medical care. We cannot emphasise too strongly that the undergraduate course in medicine should be primarily educational." *Royal Commission on Medical Education, 1968, The Todd Report.*

We learn all the time and throughout life. We learn to read and write, to ride a bike, to play games, we learn about feelings and attitudes, about pain and suffering and we learn how to make decisions.

Learning is therefore fundamental for living. Without learning, the ability to know things, to do things and to feel things, we would have no real existence. Nor could we discover new things if we did not begin with where we are now.

One of the triggers for this book was a belief that storytelling and learning are connected. That it was possible to learn some aspects of human experience and knowledge by listening to, or reading, stories. This chapter deals with the general concept of learning before moving on to the next chapter which deals more specifically with medical storytelling.

What does it mean to learn something? Learning means that we know something, can do something or feel something in a way which we were unable to do before. Learning means always beginning where we are (our present state of knowing) and the changes add to or reinforce this present state.

Learning thus covers a very wide range of actions and experiences. In medical terms it covers areas of knowledge, such as the relationships of the duodenum, the Krebs cycle, the mechanism of the action of B blockers and many many others. It considers skills such as reading an ECG, auscultating a chest, putting up an I.V. line. And finally it relates to feelings of our own and others. It is a continuous process and throughout life we change, not only our knowledge base, but our attitudes and experiences.

Some of our learning is based on formal periods in which we are in contact
with a teacher, leader or mentor who guides and facilitates our learning. In
other instances it is less formal and may well be self-directed. Much of our
learning is based on experience and in particular, on the views of others whom
we respect and who may have greater wisdom than we have. A great deal of
this latter is through the stories that others tell us, and which influence our
thinking and actions.

In medicine much of our learning, particularly of skills and attitudes is by
watching and listening to others. This "socialisation" of our learning is
particularly dependent on the hidden agenda which influences what we do,
and how we do it. We look up to, and are influenced by others in a way which
we may not even recognise, but this non-genetic aspect of behaviour change is
real (see chapter 9).

Learning of course can be both good, and bad. We can learn bad habits and
the wrong way to do things. Our factual knowledge may be incorrect and we
may not fully understand (even if it is known) the reasons for the appearance of
disease and the treatment which is appropriate. It is particularly difficult to
unlearn such bad habits, skills, and knowledge. Learning thus has no value
base associated with it.

Education on the contrary is always associated with a particular value base.
Education is a process through which learning occurs and is always for good.
Training on the other hand deals with the acquisition of particular knowledge
or skills to deal with a specific topic. It does not necessarily have a value base
(you can be trained to pick pockets). Training enables you to deal with a
particular task, education goes beyond that. The phrase "to be trained is to
have arrived, to be educated is to continue to travel", sums this up well.
(Calman & Downie, 1988).

The teacher (and the text book) have an interesting place in learning, especially
in adult learning. Teachers (and mentors) provide a guide to a particular
subject or skill. They set the context and the principles within which the subject
can be understood. They set out the main landmarks and take the student
through the major features of the topic. They define the concepts within which
the subsequent detailed work is carried out by the student.

Of course it is possible for medical students or postgraduates to learn on their own. This is indeed likely to be the most common form of learning. However, the teacher can make it easier, especially in relation to learning skills where advice, tips, supervision, feedback all assist in the process. The student learns from the master and the apprenticeship system is still an integral part of learning in medicine. In the development of a technological approach to medical teaching, and the increase in e-literacy, it is easy to forget just how important this is.

Memory is an essential part of learning. There is little point in attending a lecture, reading a textbook or scientific paper, or being taken through a surgical procedure if the process (knowledge or skill) cannot be recalled or repeated. While it is always possible to check the books or the Internet for the answer (and there are good reasons why this should be done) in practical terms the doctor has to deal with day-to-day work by remembering what to do and how to do it.

Individuals use different techniques for memorising or remembering facts, figures, skills, or attitudes. Much of this relates to repetition of the process or the knowledge which is then acquired by experience. This process is particularly relevant with a skill or procedure. But how do we remember which drug to use and what dose is most appropriate? How do we remember complex lists of facts or anatomical relationships?

One common way is by the use of mnemonics, which summarise in a generally humourous way, complex issues. The author can still remember the list and order of the cranial nerves and relationships of the lingual nerve though is unlikely to repeat them in a book of such academic distinction. Some people have visual memories and can "see" pages and diagrams in their mind and this reproduces the information readily. Others remember clinical stories and case studies which illustrate the knowledge and thus remember the correct procedure, diagnostic test or dose.

Memory builds on what we already have remembered. Memory does not occur in a vacuum and thus the process of learning is one which is continually building on existing knowledge and experience. Hence the importance (already stressed) of previous experience when learning a new subject. In educational terms this is sometimes referred to as "concept mapping". We all have existing concepts or frameworks of knowledge. These define what we know and how we act. New knowledge adds to those existing concepts and supplants them, modifies them, and may even completely change them.

Take the example of breast cancer. As an entrant to medicine the student, unless having had personal experience, is likely to know a little about cancer and what breast cancer is. The prospective student is likely to be aware that it is a common and serious illness. Early experience in medical school builds on this by an understanding of the form and function of the normal breast and subsequently its appearance in pathological conditions. All of this building and developing the concept of breast cancer and its relation to benign disease. Clinical experience adds to this and may result in a re-reading or re-thinking of the concept of the normal breast. Methods of treatment are added to the concept and as the student moves into the postgraduate field then there is an expansion in detailed knowledge and a greater emphasis on original work and research findings. The doctor may develop a particular interest in the emotions and feelings associated with breast cancer and need to develop skills in this area. All of this refining and re-interpreting the concept of breast cancer. Finally, if this is a special interest of the doctor his or her own research may change the concept for him or herself, and for others as well. This means writing a new story which will reflect a new discovery which will have come about through curiosity and listening to patient and scientific stories.

This example shows the importance of gradually building up a concept or area of knowledge and how it might be influenced by the acquisition of new knowledge or skills.

The learning environment has already been referred to briefly. Learning can occur almost anywhere and at any time. In clinical practice it can, and does. Much learning centres round particular problems (problem based learning) during which the process of solving the problem results in learning something new and different. Particularly in a postgraduate setting this is a very common experience. A new patient or a different presentation allows the re-thinking of diagnosis and management. The ability to link this to the wider information base is essential. Access to electronic information or textbooks is therefore vital and can now be done readily at ward or clinic level.

Just as important, however, is capitalising on the experience of someone who has seen the problem before and has already thought through the issue. This "learning from others" is a crucial part of medical education. However, in both instances (access to information and/or to personal experience) it is essential that this is readily available and up-to-date. If the background knowledge (in paper, electronic or personal form) is not easily accessible then the learning opportunity may be lost.

In a similar way the culture of the clinical unit, in hospital or primary care, has to be such that it encourages learning at all times and in all circumstances. It actually promotes a review of the literature and the auditing of previous cases and outcomes. This is good and effective clinical practice and the learning environment it promotes makes the practitioner more aware of new ideas and the limits of their own professional practice.

The assessment of learning. Part of being in a system of higher education is that in most circumstances it is necessary to assess the outcome of the process of learning. This is relevant at undergraduate and postgraduate levels and also in continuing professional development. The assessment of knowledge has generally been the easiest to do through essays, multiple choice test, oral examination or via Objective Structured Clinical Examination (OSCEs). These may be carried out on a regular and ongoing basis (formative testing) or at the end of a course of learning (summative assessment). Generally, before the test is set, a series of criteria are drawn up against which to mark the student (criterion referenced). In other instances, contrary to good educational practice, a fixed percentage or number are selected to pass (norm referenced) .

The assessment of skills is more difficult. It may be done on real patients, or on models or manikins. These latter are now very sophisticated and can be used to assess not only individuals, but teams of staff. In some places groups of trained patients are used with very good effect.

Most difficult of all is the assessment of attitudes and feelings. How do we assess judgement and reliability, not of the test, but of the doctor? This is generally done by the interaction between one person and another, listening and watching in real circumstances and in real time. If it is believed that appropriate attitudes are an important part of being a good doctor then we need methods for their assessment, and a definition as to what they are. As a second part of this, of course, is how such attitudes can be learned.

This is where stories, both verbal and non-verbal, become important in showing others the way things might be done. This is at the heart of the "hidden agenda" of medical education. Students, and those in training, watch others and listen and learn from them.

The curriculum should be designed, not only to cover the required content, but also to expose the student to different experiences and learning situations during which knowledge, attitudes and skills can be learned and assessed. This is not a straightforward matter, but requires great skill and the ability to modify it and change it with time and experience. Increasingly the curriculum is problem based and encourages more self-directed learning.

It is generally assumed, at least with medical students, that assessment should be carried out by doctors. This assumption should be challenged. There are many others who could and should have a legitimate interest. For example, our nursing colleagues have special skills and experience and can add greatly to the assessment process. This is being done in some medical schools at present. The second group is patients and the public. They can be very good judges of the performance of students. In some clinical skills laboratories they provide the basis of the assessment.

The final point to be made is the need for re-assessment of the doctor on a regular and on-going basis. The terms used vary from re-certification, re-accreditation to re-validation. In each the assessment is based on what has already been achieved, hence the importance of pre-registration appraisal and specialist registration as a foundation for this. From the public's point of view this is essential if trust and confidence in the profession are to be maintained.

Theories of Learning. So far the discussion has been based on some general aspects of learning. In this section a more systematic view will be taken and some of the major theories about how we learn will be considered. There are a wide range of books on this subject (see for example "The Theory and Practice of Learning" P. Jarvis, J Holford, and C Griffin, 1998, Kogan Page).

Some general issues. Much has changed in the world of education over the last few decades. Life - long learning and continuing professional development are now high on the agenda. There has also been a significant shift from teacher centred learning to student centred learning. This shift is important and is reflected in most medical school curricula. More people are now in the educational system, especially at the level of higher education. This has raised relevant issues of selection for medical courses and the need, not only for fairness in the process, but for an explicit statement of how the process operates. There has also been a debate on the language used; education, training, competence, vocational, practical. It sometimes seems as if these words are not related. In medical terms, as we have already noted, there is a distinction between education and training, though both are appropriate, and both relevant. In a similar way, vocational and practical are both terms which are widely used. The terms distance and open learning are of interest in medicine and with the development of e-learning this has made these concepts even more important.

Two issues are of special interest in medicine. The first of these is in the rapidly changing knowledge base. The pace of change is phenomenal, and is difficult to keep up with. The implications for medical education are thus considerable. How do we ensure that students have access to this information, and that the information itself is validated? How can we test students on such a changing base? What role do manikins and computer simulations have? Will they replace the patient for the learning of skills and procedures? How will we ensure that students have the skills to access and use the information? Patients will be using the web, doctors cannot be left behind. The educational methodology and the pedagogy meet to be able to respond to this. With the increasing use of such technology, will face to face contact be phased out? Will we still listen to the stories of others, and will the apprenticeship system in which the young doctor learns from the master be a thing of the past? Hopefully this will not happen and the technology will be used as a way of supporting learning, rather than an end in itself. This will be discussed more fully later in this chapter.

The second aspect is the social environment and context in which learning occurs. There are considerable changes in the demography of the population and in social attitudes and values. The world is smaller, and the use of the term "globalisation" is increasingly used (Giddens, 1999). But it is more than this. The policy context is also changing. The university and higher education system is changing rapidly. The National Health Service, a remarkable organisation, is being, and has been, radically altered, and the professions are re-thinking their values and standards. In the midst of all of this doctors need to be able to continue to learn the practice of medicine and to meet these changes head on.

The next section reviews some of the major theories of learning. In this part of the chapter the word student is used in a generic sense to cover all those who wish to learn; old or young, formal or informal, undergraduate or postgraduate, freshman or vice-chancellor. Those at the top of the tree also need to continue to learn and be fellow students.

Behaviourist approaches. The two key names in this field are Pavlov and Skinner. In essence the proposition behind this theory is that "learning is any more or less permanent change in behaviour which is the result of experience". Thus, the outcome is always measured in terms of behaviour change and is based on the kind of stimulus response experiments carried out by Pavlov on dogs. The person becomes "conditioned" to behave in a particular way. In practical terms this may occur by "trial and error" in which the individual learns the best way to behave. This, in terms of patient care would be inappropriate, though the process of learning in this way is valuable in itself. The learning, of course, can be modified by the teacher who guides the process and assists the student. The second way in which the behaviourist approach can be effected is by set objectives, in order that the student knows what behaviour is expected of him or her. For example, "By the end of this chapter the reader should be able to list the major theories of education". Or, "By the end of this chapter the reader should be able to give four examples of the use of stories in learning". These are valuable tools, but it must be obvious that there are some limitations to the process. For example it is easy to set objectives which are easily measured, and the approach works best where there are clear outcomes. The third option is to take this approach even further and to set competencies to be achieved. For example, by the end of the medical course all students should be able to take a history, record a blood pressure and make a diagnosis of most common diseases. At the postgraduate level it might be to demonstrate a specific skill in a procedure or management. Such competencies allow the curriculum to be defined more clearly and for them to be regularly assessed over the years in processes such as re-validation. The limitations are again clear. As the knowledge base changes so will the required competencies, and there are some high level activities such as judgement and curiosity which cannot be readily assessed in this way.

Cognitivist theories. Such theories are based on the way in which the mind develops and the key name here is Piaget. His work was mainly on children and related development to the capacity to learn. The theory concerns thinking and reflection and understanding, and is not therefore based in reflex responses to stimuli. Brain work is required. It relates to our experiences and how we interpret them and use them.

Social learning. Much of our learning takes place not just as individuals, but in a social context, and indeed this is where the stories of others have a particular role. We listen and learn from where we work, and who our friends and colleagues happen to be. We are influenced by all around us, and the groups with whom we associate. We conform and learn the rules of the group. This is essentially, in medical terms, the process of socialisation into the profession.

There is a further dimension to this, and is well recognised by those who have moved away from a clinical unit and returned, having gone to learn a new technique or procedure and returned to the ward or clinic. In favourable circumstances it will be possible to introduce the new procedure whatever it is. In practice it may be very difficult, The social milieu is against it. It's too much to change, and it wouldn't work anyway. There must be many doctors, and other health care professionals who have tried to do something new and been thwarted by the social norm. Change and organisational learning is difficult.

Experiential learning. In one sense all learning is based on experience. Kant, in "The Critique of Pure Reason" says that "all our knowledge begins with experience, there can be no doubt". It is very relevant in medicine where a direct exposure to a problem and its management can have a real impact. Watching, listening, doing and reflecting on a real problem is very powerful. Such experiences change our perceptions of problems and how to handle them. As many of the attributes of the doctor are related to attitudes our prejudices are important. Experiences can be formative and change our perceptions and so we need to have our own feelings, skills and knowledge constantly challenged. It would be difficult to be a good doctor without experience of real patients and their problems, and listening to their stories and their response to illness.

Much of what has been discussed in the previous sections can be summarised in the educational cycle. Different words are used for this and it is just as relevant to clinical audit and to the management of almost any problem. It begins with **assessment** of the problem or of the learning needs. This is followed by a period of **planning**, which takes account of these needs and sets objectives to be achieved. The third phase in the cycle is **implementation**, in which the student puts into practice the plan which has been developed. Finally there is the phase of **evaluation**, where the process and outcomes are reviewed, and the whole cycle started again. Readers with a keen eye will have noted that the initial letters of the words of this cycle end up with the mnemonic, **a pie**. Another bit of useless information.

A consideration of such a cycle leads to a discussion of the use of contracts in education and learning. In this process the learner and the teacher or mentor begin with the assessment and set out the key areas to be tackled. Part of the contract will be delivered by the student (attend certain seminars, write essays, see patients, etc) and part of it by the teacher or organisation (library facilities, supervision, access to patients etc). The contract is then reviewed at intervals. Thus the diagnosis of learning needs is at the heart of the learning process. To use that well known phrase again, learning begins from where the learner starts, not where the teacher thinks the student is. Learning contracts are being used increasingly in medicine.

In medical terms, much learning is self-directed and is a result of a patient problem which requires greater understanding, or a subject of curiosity which is stimulated and needs to be looked into. Problem based learning is a powerful way of stimulating active learning and involvement of the student. Practical examples, hands on experiments in laboratories, real patients, can make all the difference to learning. The skills (now called key skills in the jargon) of working on problems and in teams, analysing data, collating it and presenting it to others is an important part of the educational process. The availability of the Internet can only add to the range of materials to be used by students, of any age.

Educational research. This has always been the poor relation of the research world. It always seems to be difficult to fund research projects, as they fall between several stools. What research has been done in adult education and in the higher education system has helped greatly to see and do things differently. The research is not difficult to find, though one wonders how many doctors regularly look, for example, at the journal, "Medical Education". Some of it relies on "clinical trial" type methodology, but much is of a different sort.

One interesting technique, for example, is the use of stories in research. The Critical Incident Technique, developed with airline pilots, asks about memorable incidents, good and bad, which have affected the performance of the job (Flanagan, 1954). These stories are then collected together and analysed and from this key areas which are performed well or badly are identified. This can then be fed back into the system, and the teaching and learning improved. As one example of this a study of pre-registration house officers was carried out using this technique to identify strengths and weaknesses (Calman and Donaldson,1991).

Other educational research using stories is well recorded (for example, McEwan and Egan,1995, Nelson, 1997, Greenhalgh and Hurwitz, 1998) and thus stories may be used both for learning and for assessment, and also as a research tool.

E-learning and e-literacy. The extraordinary rapidity with which the Internet and its associated technology is developing provides another dimension to education and learning. It is now possible with a few clicks to gain access to the most up-to-date information in the world. Subject to a few small technical issues this can be accessed almost anywhere. How are we to use this information revolution to improve and expand the ways in which we learn? This will remain an important topic in education for some time to come. The comparison with the introduction of books centuries ago is interesting. There was a fear that a single book (or e-learning source) would be all that would be required to cover a subject. There would be one information source on astronomy, or anatomy. However this is not what happened. Those who read the books wanted to write a different one and to put forward new ideas and ways of thinking. As new discoveries were made so the books had to change, and this will be made all the more easy because of the technology. But still those who wanted to learn went to others who would pass on their learning to them. The personal contact between two minds was important, and it is likely to be so, especially at the higher end of the educational system. There are those who will write the learning material, and others who will use it.

Educational leadership. It has been assumed in this chapter that leadership is required if the process is to be effective and have direction. However, it is such an important topic that it is highlighted here. It takes us back to heroes and legends, and our own mentors and teachers. They guided and stimulated, enthused and cajoled. They helped choose the speciality we entered because of their dedication and competence and by the personal interest they took in us. We need such people who not only provide a first class clinical service, but develop and maintain the continuity of the profession. They do take an interest and do look after our well being. One of the definitions of education is "the process by which values are transmitted from one generation to another". They cared, and still do care, about the profession and the future of their own speciality. They wanted it to do well and looked out for those who might take it forward.

One of the starting points of this book was the work of Howard Gardner in his book "Leading Minds" (1995) where, beginning from an educational background, he looked at leadership and the link to storytelling. He concludes that the two are related and that good leaders and good teachers tell good stories. Many of our own personal experiences would support this.

This leads nicely into a discussion on the role of storytelling in medical education.

STORYTELLING IN MEDICAL EDUCATION. It should be obvious that this discussion is simply a sub-set of the use of stories in education generally. We learn through stories and doctors are no exception. In theoretical terms the writings on Brunner and others (see Brunner 1986, 1990) shed some light on the processes involved. There are two types of learning proposed. The first concerns the logical processing of information and knowledge, typically from a book or journal or from a formal lecture. The aim is to transmit factual knowledge. This is essential for the doctor. She must know what to do and how to do it. The second is the transmission of feelings and attitudes. This can best be done in other ways, notably through stories. The two areas overlap considerably, but the two positions can be recognised. The teaching of skills is likely to require a mixture of the two. The important point is that both are necessary, they are not in competition, but complementary.

Related to this is the need to connect the anecdote with the evidence. This book is not a plea for storytelling in medicine to be the only way forward, far from it. But it does see it as relevant. Just as we need the evidence base so we need a source of inspiration for the more human aspects of medical practice. To divorce the two would be inappropriate. The power of the story is that it connects the individual patient with the rest of the world literature. It takes the doctor from an anecdote to a whole book of stories collected and analysed and ready to be compared and contrasted. Putting the two together may be where learning begins, and the mixture is essential.

The settings. Stories can be used in a wide variety of ways and in very different settings. These might include.

The formal setting. This would include lectures and seminars and other forms of formal presentation. Stories can be included as individual patient histories, or by videos or on the Internet. Cartoons may be used to stimulate interest and to expand and exemplify a particular point. The story may help the student to remember the factual issue and be able to recall it more readily. It might be supposed that it would be impossible to teach biochemistry or pharmacology with stories but the following example, by the author, on chemotherapeutic agents in cancer management, delivered at a conference on methotrexate, shows that it is possible. Other forays in this genre have been in skin pathology and ophthalmology.

In praise of Methotrexate
I want to tell a story of some anti-cancer drugs,
So sit back, charge your glasses, and pin back both your lugs.
It all began with Ehrlich, of "magic bullet" fame,
Back in the 1890s when science was just a game.
He synthesised an alkylator ethylenimine,
The first true cytotoxic the world had ever seen.
A space of forty years elapsed, until in time of war
The ship, the John F Harvey sank down in Bari Harbor.
Aboard this ship was mustard gas its effects the Bard recites

Made many of the men right sick and dropped their leucocytes.
The medic, Alexander, had a flash of inspiration
That clinical benefit might result when the white count showed elevation.
So Goodman and Gilman and Dougherty from the field of Academia
Assessed the use of mustard in childhood and adult leukemia.
And so the scene is set, Sidney Farber's on the stage.
The drug was Methotrexate and chemotherapy came of age.
Aminopterin was first, or so the Bard relates,
Both compounds being active as synthetic antifolates.
The drug is given orally or by the intravenous route,
Intramuscularly, intrathecally, which ever one will suit.
In pharmacokinetics fit a three compartment system.
It has three half lives in venous blood, but I do not wish to list them.
Its mechanism of action, its biochemical pharmacology
Have been described for many years and are like dogma in oncology.
Methotrexate acts, or so the Bard oft says
On a critical enzyme molecule, dihydrofolate reductase.
It has a very high affinity 10-8 or more
And inhibits the conversion of FH2 to FH4.
Enzyme action is inhibited at micromolar concentration,
Always of course assuming adequate drug penetration.

Other enzymes are important like carboxypeptidase,
Hepatic aldehyde oxidase and thymidylate synthetase.
Thymidine kinase is another catalyst.
The others have much longer names I will not even list.
Its action on the cell cycle is really quite terrific
Like some other antimetabolites Methotrexate is S-phase specific.
Methotrexate does exist in many different states
And currently the interests is in polyglutamates.
There are monoglu's and diglu's and glu's to the power N,
Their significance however is quite beyond my ken.
To measure Methotrexate is not an easy task.
Which methods are the best ones do I hear you ask?
Well there's GLC, HPLC and radioimmunoassay,
And EMIT kits of course which are actually rather classy.
Some techniques at first were really rather primitive

And couldn't even measure the 7-hydroxy derivative.
The side effects of Methotrexate must not be forgotten.
Mucositis is perhaps the worst in fact it's rather rotten.
Renal damage may result and can accentuate toxicity,
Hepatic damage can occur when its given with some chronicity.
Sore eyes can be a problem and reddened conjunctiva,
Methotrexate is secreted in the tears and in saliva.
One side effect however which has not been documented
Is car-cin-o-genesis which makes one quite contented.
So far the evidence suggests, and the Bard has not heard rumours,
That Methotrexate, given long term, does not cause second tumours.

Before I bring this rambling verse to a necessary close,
I must mention Methotrexate given in mega dose.
Instead of 15 migs. we now use 15 gram
And such doses can be repeated, in fact ad nauseam.
Folinic acid rescue is the secret of success,
Without old Leucovarin we'd be in quite a mess.
Well I'm getting tired now and on my feet I teeter,
But before I end this rhyme I should like to change the metre
Because

You can flatten them with platinum,
Get big cell kill from fluorouracil
Be a medicine man with melphalan
Keep things pristine with vincristine.
Shout with glee with 6MP.
Quite amaze with asparginase.
Be the boss with cyclophos.
Never be alone with prednisone.
But don't touch custard after mustard.
Play to win with Doxorubicin.
But you can fix it with Methotrexate.

The classic work of Sir Zachary Cope (1962) on the diagnosis of the acute abdomen in rhyme shows how well this can be done. The next challenge is the Krebs cycle.

The clinical setting. This is an obvious opportunity for the telling of stories, from patients and from experience. They can be used to amplify and develop a presentation of a clinical problem. Patient stories are the clearest example of this. There is however the doctor to doctor communication about patients. This happens all the time, advice is sought and given. It's sometimes easier and faster, even with the Internet, to ask a colleague for help and an opinion. It presents a clear learning situation. The informal meetings amongst doctors are thus very valuable. It encourages discussion and the sharing of views. It acts as a means of audit and of standard setting. Postgraduate meetings are just as valuable for this function as the formal presentation.

From the public. The public is an important source of stories about themselves and the services they have used. Tell someone in the holiday hotel that you are a doctor and the stories begin. Even more interesting is to sit in a clinic or an Accident and Emergency Department and listen to what happens and observe the stories being told in front of your eyes. One of the most powerful educational experiences of the author was in the setting up of a series of patient groups for cancer patients. In an informal setting as friends rather than as patient-doctor the real feelings surface and the service you thought was excellent is clearly capable of improvement. Getting close to patients is not a bad thing if it helps you understand their feelings and concerns.

SOME END PIECES

The discussion in the previous sections has set out the conventional ways of looking at teaching and learning and the role of storytelling. This section picks up a few issues which don't fit neatly into this picture. The first of these will be the subject of a full chapter later in the book and this concerns the concept of the contagious theory of behaviour change. In this concept it is proposed that individuals, through stories and their behaviour, can change others. They transmit ideas and attitudes. This concept argues for close contact, though this may not need to be face to face, between individuals, as other models may be used. There are, in addition to this topic, a number of other issues which need further debate.

The apprenticeship model. In the discussion and debate on medical education, and in the flurry of reports and proposals, the power of the apprenticeship model has sometimes been lost. Yet it fits well with the general proposition that we learn many things from others, by watching and listening what they do. The apprenticeship works in real time and with real people and patients. There is often no time for the considered opinion and a review of the literature, the decision has to be made there and then. The processes by which such decisions are made can be watched and observed. As new information becomes available during the management of the patient so the decisions are reviewed and re-assessed. This is a very formative experience in dealing with difficult problems. It shows how senior doctors work, how they interact with the wider caring team, and the patient and family. In the reforms of higher specialist training in the UK the importance of this aspect was never in doubt. What was proposed was that the process of education over the period of specialist training would be more structured and associated with regular review of performance and feedback. This is entirely consistent with the use of the apprenticeship model. This discussion leads directly into the next subject, that of the role of judgement and wisdom in medicine.

Judgement and wisdom in medicine. In most professions those who exercise judgement and wisdom are highly prized, and in medicine the same is true (Downie and Macnaughton, 2000). In almost all hospitals there is a "wise" physician or surgeon to whom difficult problems are sent. They are often generalists and have wide experience. They have been the bedrock of first class clinical practice and teaching. The question for this book is how we can ensure that such individuals are replicated and that their experience is not lost. Part of the solution is in listening to their stories, watching the way in which decisions are made and problems resolved. This cannot be taught by setting objectives, and re-structuring the medical course. It is only likely to occur with much higher order thinking. It is important, however, that we recognise its value and try to understand the processes behind it. How do we gain wisdom? This has been the subject of discussion for generations. It goes beyond and is deeper than knowledge, though this is clearly relevant, and has something to do with the individual being having sufficient self-knowledge to deal with problems. Much of this wisdom may come from experience outside of medical practice.

Curiosity. This is another of the words which are used regularly in medical education. It can be defined as an "eager desire to know, inquisitiveness." The General Medical Council encourages students to exhibit this attribute as follows,

"Attitudinal Objectives. Approaches to learning that are based on curiosity and the exploration of knowledge rather than its passive acquisition, and that will be retained throughout life."

As a concept it appears frequently in articles and books. But what does it mean? Can it be taught? How do you measure it?

It is clearly an active concept, the learner has to do something, and show the attributes of eagerness, of inquisitiveness, and a desire to know more. It is a concept associated with exploration, adventure, discovery and hypothesis testing. It requires both observation using all of the senses and the need to check all that has already been discovered by checking the literature. If this is what it means, how can, or could, we test it? Perhaps by reviewing library and Internet skills, assessing interest and enthusiasm, by ensuring that students have opportunities to test their own curiosity. This is regularly done by project work, laboratory assignments, "fieldwork" and clinical placements in different units. The special study modules would be a good example of this.

It is clearly important that doctors have this ability to be curious, and that in so doing can improve the treatment or understanding of disease.

Epiphany. This is an old concept which is now increasingly used in educational terms and especially in relation to story telling (Hawkins, 1997). An epiphanic experience relates to the sudden discovery or insight into some aspect of nature. It is of particular interest in issues around innovation and creativity. The student suddenly "sees" the answer, or the way to carry out a task. It is an important aspect of learning when the pieces all seem to fit together at last. It is also of interest in ethical issues and it is here that stories can be used to open eyes to a special problem. This will be discussed more fully in chapter 8.

SOME CONCLUSIONS

This chapter has taken a broad view of education and learning and has specifically described the role of storytelling in this context. The power of the story has been emphasised, but its complementary relationship with information and knowledge acquisition has been acknowledged. The two are not in competition, and the anecdote and the evidence base need to be connected. The medical student of today needs anatomy, physiology and pathology as never before. We need to be assured that young doctors understand and can take forward the new advances in genetics and molecular biology. They need to be alert to new clinical advances and the results of clinical trials. And on the other hand be concerned, considerate and compassionate for their patients. Both are required if the doctor is to be a rounded and whole person. There is always a danger that in the development of educational programmes the higher level skills such as judgement and wisdom may be lost. These, however, are critical faculties and need to be understood. The apprenticeship model linked to a structured educational programme puts the two together. Finally the issue of insight into problems and to finding solutions, the epiphanic experience is an important one and again we need to understand it better.

REFERENCES

Brunner,J. Acts of Meaning. 1990, Harvard University Press. Cambridge. Mass.

Brunner,J. Actual Minds, Possible Words. 1986. Harvard University Press. Cambridge Mass.

Calman, K.C. and Donaldson,M. The pre-registration house officer year: a critical incident study, 1991, Medical Education. 25, 51-59.

Calman,K.C, and Downie, R.S. Education and training in medicine.1988 Medical Education, 22, 488-91.

Cope,Z. The Acute Abdomen in Rhyme. 1962. H.K.Lewis, London.

Downie, R.S. and Macnaughton, J. Clinical Judgement. Evidence in Practice. 2000. Oxford University Press.

Flanagan, J.C. The critical incident technique. 1954. Psychological Bulletin, 51, 327-58

Gardner, H. Leading Minds. An Anatomy of Leadership. 1995. Harper Collins, London.

Giddens. A. Runaway World. 1999, Profile Books, London.

Greenhalgh, T, and Hurwitz, B. Narrative based medicine. Dialogue and discourse in clinical practice. 1998. Brit. Med. J Publishing Group, London.

Hawkins, A.H. Medical ethics and the epiphanic dimension of narrative. 1997. In, Stories and Their Limits. Ed H.L.Nelson. Routledge, New York and London.

Jarvis,P, Holford,J, and Griffin,C. The Theory and Practice of Learning. 1998, Kogan Page, London.

McEwan, H and Egan, K, Narrative in Teaching Learning and Research. 1995. Teachers College Press, Columbia University, New York.

Nelson, H.L. Editor. Stories and Their Limits.1997, Routledge, New York and London.

6. From Aphorism to Cyberspace: Medical Stories in Writing. Big Stories and Wee Ones.

"Life is short, and the art long. Opportunity is elusive, experiment is dangerous, judgement difficult. It is not enough for the physician to do what is necessary, but the patient and the attendants must do their part as well, and the circumstances must be favourable." *The Aphorisms of Hippocrates.*

Medical stories come in very different shapes and forms and it might be assumed that fiction would be the preferred way of illustrating the range. But, as has been described in the Introduction, much has already been written on this theme. Doctors as writers, and doctors in literature, books about illness and disease, or of suffering and pain. This chapter takes a different line and discusses the stories written by doctors in a more medical mode, that of aphorisms, case histories, log books and textbooks, and more recently the use of the internet and computing. As less has been written on the literature around medical students, this will be the one exception.

APHORISMS. Aphorisms have been the traditional way in which medical wisdom has been transmitted through the generations. These "wee" stories are short and easily remembered phrases or statements which could be referred to in times of need to provide a basis for both diagnosis and management. The earliest of these can be found in the works of the Greek physicians, of whom Hippocrates is the most obvious. The aphorisms in his works are remarkable for their depth and breadth and would have provided a ready source of learning the rudiments of medicine. Take the following.

"Desperate cases need the most desperate remedies."

"When a disease has attained the crisis, or when the crisis has just passed, do not disturb the patient with innovation in treatment..."

"Rest as soon as there is pain is a great restorative in all disturbances of the body."
"To the love of his profession the physician should add a love of humanity."

For some, however, the evidence base seems lacking.
"People who lisp are especially liable to prolonged diarrhoea."

There have been collections of such aphorisms made over the years. They are fascinating and full of humour and wisdom, though not always associated with a clinical trial of sufficient power to make the case properly. Bean (W.B. Bean, 1962, The Aphorisms of Latham, 1962, The Prairie Press, Iowa City) describes the wisdom of Peter Latham a 19th century physician at St Bartholomew's Hospital in London. He notes a fascinating phrase to describe aphorisms. They are seen to be:

"Burrs that stick in the mind"

We remember them, and recall them when we need them.

For example here are some of the collected aporisms of the Mayo brothers, Charles and William, brought together by Willius (F.A.Willius, Aphorisms of Dr Charles and Dr William Mayo, 1951, Whiting Press Inc. Rochester, Minnesota.)

"Carry out the two fundamental surgical requirements: see what you are doing and leave a dry field."

"Judgement is a great asset; it makes the diagnostician and the surgeon both supermen."

"The writer of textbooks should have a ready imagination, and he should understand the child's mind."

"Once you start studying medicine you never get through with it."

"The university, through it's organised intelligence, controls the future."

Many such sayings were collected by James Alexander Lindsey, Professor of Medicine at Queen's University in Belfast. (J.L.Lindsey, Medical Aphorisms and

Axioms, and Clinical Memoranda. 1923, H.K. Lewis, London.) Again they reveal the ways in which doctors have thought and acted over the centuries.

"Rest and abstinence are the best of all remedies, and abstinence alone cures without any danger." *Celsus.*

"The sick should be the doctor's books." *Paracelcus.*

"Never believe what a patient tells you his doctor has said." *William Jenner*.

"The trouble with most doctors is, not that they don't know enough, but that they don't see enough." *Dominic Corrigan.*

"Always examine the bases of the lungs in cases of obscure illness."

"The asthmatic should go supperless to bed."

"A localised tuberculosis infection is only a skirmish, such as is constantly going on at the frontiers of the empire." *W. Osler.*

"Tell a cardiac patient to find out what he can do and do it; tell him to find out what he cannot do and never do it." *Clifford Allbutt.*

"The treatment of high blood-pressure is a régime, not a drug." *Huchard.*

"Tremor is a succession of similar movements; chorea is a succession of different movements." *Hughlings Jackson.*

"A slight ailment often promotes longevity." *Oliver Wendell Holmes.*

"The physician who cannot cure chlorosis should retire from the practice of his profession." *W. Osler.*

"An attack of psoriasis is a certificate of good health." *Jonathan Hutchinson.*

"Sunlight has a marked analgesic effect." *H. Gauvain.*

John Hunter, when challenged regarding an inconsistency in his teaching, replied: "Perhaps I did say so and so. I hope I grow wiser every year".

"In the field of experiment chance only favours the mind that is prepared." *Pasteur.*

"Without hypotheses there is no useful observation." *Charles Darwin.*

"By the neglect of the study of the humanities, which has been far too general, the profession of medicine loses a very precious quality." *W. Osler.*

Others followed and it was not uncommon to have books of aphorisms by some of the most distinguished medical people of their generation and they have been reproduced here as the source books are sometimes difficult to find. Others to browse through would include

"Mould's Medical Anecdotes", *Omnibus Edition, 1996, Institute of Physics Publishing, Bristol*

"Aphorisms from his Bedside" *Teachings and Writings of William Osler, 1961, Second Printing.*

"Medical Quotes. A thematic dictionary." *Edited by J Daintith and A Isaacs, 1989, Market House Books Ltd, Aylesbury.*

In 1977 Sir Rodney Smith (later Lord Smith) reviewed in his Hitchener Lecture (J. Roy. Army. Med. Cps 123, 57 - 64) some masters of the surgical aphorism and it makes fascinating reading.

And they remain important even to this day. The aphorism "Remember the man with the glass eye and the big liver" refers to a patient with malignant melanoma of the eye, which had been enucleated, and which had spread to the liver. The author was well aware of this as a medical student, but as a clinical oncologist, the first time such a patient was seen with the glass eye and the big liver, the message came back immediately. Heard as a student and instantly remembered.

There is much history in aphorisms and a study of them reveals how medical thinking has changed over the generations. As is commented on elsewhere in this book, "The history of medicine is the re-classification of disease". These brief comments by the giants of their age show how far we have come and how far we have still to go.

MEDICAL NOTES

The second phase of the development of medical writing was the use of medical case notes. These are generally very carefully written and can give great insights into the illnesses of the time and the treatments available. They are often written in great detail and with enormous care. Here are some illustrations, and again it would be difficult not to begin with Hippocrates. This case is from Epidemics Book I and is discussed in considerable depth.

"Herophon suffered from a high fever. Stools small with temesmus at first; afterwards he passed thin bilious matter rather frequently. He could not sleep, urine dark and thin.

Early on the fifth day, became deaf, all the symptoms were more pronounced, the spleen became enlarged, the hypochondrium contracted; he passed a small quantity of dark matter from his bowels. He was delirious.

Sixth day: babbling at random, at night sweating, became cold remained delirious.

Seventh day: became cold, thirsty, out of his mind. Regained control of his mind during the night and slept.

Eighth day: fever, the spleen reduced in size, and he was wholly lucid. He felt pain at first in the groin on the same side as the spleen, later on pains in the calves of both legs. Passed a comfortable night. Urine of better colour with a slight sediment.

Ninth day: sweating, the crisis was reached and the fever left him.

On the fifth day after this a relapse occurred. The spleen immediately enlarged; high fever, deafness again. On the third day of the relapse, the spleen became reduced, the deafness less; pain in the legs; sweating during the night. A crisis was reached about the seventeenth day. There was no delirium during the relapse."

Another illustration of this type of case description comes from the works of Dr John Hall, the son-in-law of William Shakespeare. Take this memorable one.

Observ. LXXI

"John Nason of Stratford upon Avon, Barber, aged 40, always after meat suffered most bitter Pains of the Stomach, as also cruel Misery in the Loins, so that he seldom had any sleep at nights, was entering into the yellow jaundice; his urine was thin, red, and the crown yellow and frothy. ℞ our emetick infusion Zi. It gave six vomits, and four stools. The following day, ℞ Horehound, Hops, Roots of Bugloss, Elicampane, and Eupatory. Rhubarb grossly sliced, Wood of aloes. Boil them all in three pints of White wine, till the third part be wasted; after strain it without expression; to the straining add the juice of goose dung half a pint. Of this he took Ziii with white sugar. This quantity he drunk betimes in the morning. And thus in a few days space he was cured, and well coloured." In John Hall, Man and Physician. by Harriet Joseph, 1976, printed in the United States.

No wonder he got better.

As a further example, which illustrates the negative side of story telling, here are some quotes from a book by John Pattison, written in 1866. (J. Pattison, Cancer its Nature and Successful and Comparatively Painless Treatment, H. Turner, London 1866). Pattison was a nephew of Granville Sharpe Pattison, Professor of surgery and anatomy in Glasgow and who emigrated to the United States of America. He sets out a new way of treating cancer, though despite reading the book several times it is difficult to know precisely what the treatment was. The book is full of anecdotes and letters of support from patients. It contains passages which are highly critical of other doctors, and there is at the end no real evidence on which to make any judgements as to the value of the treatment. Judge for yourself.

"Ulcerated cancer of the right breast." *Camberwell, January 11th 1865.*

Dear Sir, Feeling conscientiously bound to acknowledge your skill and kindness in the treatment of my case, I send you the following statement of its progress from the commencement to the present time.

About five years ago, at the age of 60, I discovered a lump in my right breast, for which I had medical attendance for more than a year; but the gentleman concealing the fact of its being cancer prevented my seeking further advice until it had assumed a malignant form. Then I consulted Mr Paget of Harewood Place who recommended an immediate operation, but as he could not even promise a cure, I was induced to consult Mr Bowman of Clifford Street who not concurring in the opinion of Mr Paget, I consulted......I allowed three months to elapse, when hearing of the most satisfactory results in many cases under your care, induced me to consult you, and I can thankfully testify to the benefit I derived from your judicious treatment.....From the great relief I experienced from the removal of the diseased parts, completely relieving me from all pain, without causing me injury to my general health."
And again,

"Case942 Mrs W aged 47 years.

This lady first observed a small lump in her right breast in the early part of the year 1857. She immediately came up to London and consulted Dr Marsden the chief surgeon of the Brompton Cancer Hospital. When he first saw it he said it was not far enough advanced for an operation but gave her the following prescription, meant I suppose to bring the disease into a fit state for operation by the knife.....The following November Dr Marsden pronounced the breast to be ripe for the knife, and he accordingly operated. The internal treatment after the operation was merely an increased quantity of carbonate of soda.....The too celebrated lead and oil liniment was also ordered.....No experienced surgeon will be surprised to learn that she grew slowly worse. She persevered in using the liniment for more than a year; what was the result? Why what exactly any man who has got a tyro's knowledge of his profession would have predicted from using such a lotion for so long; not only did the disease increase, but she also suffered from lead poisoning.....The lady came to see me on the 29th June 1859, suffering from ulcerated cancer.....and from lead poisoning accompanied by paralysis. And now I have succeeded in removing all traces of lead, and have nearly cured her cancerous disease."

How he did this he unfortunately does not say.

William Osler was the doyen of physicians at the turn of the 19th and 20th centuries. In a book entitled "Lectures on the Diagnosis of Abdominal Tumours" published in 1895 (Henry Kimpton, London) while he was still Professor of Medicine at Johns Hopkins Hospital, Baltimore, he describes in very great detail the patients he saw, diagnosed and managed. Here is a very short extract.

"Case XXIV. Large, massive tumour in the epigastric and upper umbilical regions. Patrick C. Harness, maker, aged 56 years, admitted April 15th, complaining of weakness and a lump in the left side.
Family history is negative; father died in an accident; mother, cause unknown, aged 55 years.

Patient has never been a very strong man; was hurt when a lad by falling off a load of hay; rheumatism in1876. He has always been rather pale; lived a sedentary life; has not been a heavy drinker; never had venereal disease. Within the last year he has lost between twenty and thirty pounds in weight.

Present illness began about a year ago...."

The patient seen a century ago comes alive and you want to read on.

Written case reports, as opposed to those delivered orally, thus record the details of an individual patient, in order that they can be reviewed and presented to the widest possible audience. In some instances such letters and case reports can herald a new disease or syndrome, HIV infection for example came to light in this way. Case reports of this illness appeared first before the larger series pointed to a new disease process. They are illustrative of clinical problems from which lessons can be learned. They are also of great historical interest recording symptoms and patterns of illness.

Case reports are a regular feature of medical journals and as this section of the book was being written the Lancet of the 18th December 1999 came through the letter box. In it was a fascinating case report by U.S. Bjornsdottir and D Smith. (Lancet 354, 1999, 2130.) It describes the poisoning of an African religious leader by organophosphates placed in his clothing. This was medical detective work at its most fascinating, and a memorable case history. The journals are full of them. Vignettes and stories of especial value highlighting problems and solutions. It is to be hoped that they continue to bring medicine alive and immediate.

On the same day the author looked at the textbooks he used as a medical student. The first two found were "Practical Paediatric Problems" by J.H Hutchison (Lloyd-Luke 1964) and "A Short Practice of Surgery" by Bailey and Love, 12th Edition, Lewis, London, 1962. In both, rather surprisingly, as it had been forgotten, there were written a series of case notes on small pieces of paper (the page would never have been written on!) to amplify the text. Some of the clinical problems could even be remembered, such is the power of stories, 30 years on.

The case history or log book therefore is not an end in itself, but a means by which new knowledge can be distributed and which might also lead to a greater understanding of a disease or illness. The exegesis of the story matters, and there needs to be time for reflection, discussion and interpretation.

Log books and diaries. Use is increasingly being made of log books and diaries in medical education. They are used to record clinical experience and can provide a mechanism of reflecting on practice and management. They can also be used to assess the range of experience of the trainee and the level of skill. Collected together and compared to the literature generally they can be an effective means of learning and research.

These observations on case notes and log books lead naturally into the next section of this chapter, in which these case histories are put together and organised into textbooks to present a wider perspective on a medical topic.

THE TEXTBOOK. The medical textbook is a very special form of medical writing and story telling. The great medical textbooks have had a profound influence on medical practice. They have guided generations of students and doctors. What do they still have to offer, and can they compete with the Internet and the CD-rom? William Osler had thought about this, and the following quotation comes from the Preface to the 9th Edition of Osler's "Principles and Practice of Medicine." (B Appleton and Co, New York, 1921, a personal copy) written by Thomas McCrae. He makes the point that "The Textbook of Medicine was one of the great interests in Osler's life. Osler said that it brought him "mind to mind" with members of the profession on many parts of the world." What a justification for writing a textbook, to bring you "mind to mind" with your readers.

In addition to containing lots of information about the subject, textbooks provide a way of organising medical information which is individual to the author. Reading a textbook provides an insight into the thinking of a person (or more recently a group of persons) and how they view the subject. They provide the introduction to a whole new world and explore the nature of the subject.

Consider the following. You are asked to write a textbook on your favourite clinical subject. How do you begin? How many chapters or sections should there be?
Do you use case studies, illustrations or figures? Will it just be a collection of facts and figures, or will there be a theme and an objective? Will you begin with structure and then proceed to normal function and then pathology, or will you begin with the problem? How much will you assume from your readers? Will you operate in an integrated way, problem based with questions and answers? Your response to these questions, and many others of course, will determine the outcome and will define your view of the subject. It will emphasise what is important to you and your own experience. As a final test check your own medical textbooks you used as a student and see if you would organise it in the same way now.

Some classic textbooks. It is not difficult to find examples of textbooks which have stood the test of time. Osler's Textbook of Medicine, Muir's Textbook of Pathology, Gray's Anatomy, and many others. These classic texts lasted for some generations and provided the guidebook which the student required. They were personal and represented a particular view. This indeed is their value. They provide a critical view at a moment in time of the knowledge available. Textbooks must always (particularly at the present time) be out of date. Knowledge moves too fast for them to keep up with the literature in the journals and the Internet. But that is not their purpose. It is to introduce you, the student, to a subject (often to a very advanced level) and provide a mechanism and a framework within which you can place and absorb new knowledge.

The organisation of knowledge, like a good story, requires considerable skill and experience. How a subject comes together, how it is presented and codified is critical. That's what good textbooks do. They take a complex subject and simplify it and create ways into the topic which are understandable and logical. They are not simply lists of clinical trials and meta-analyses. They are much more.

Consider a second option. You have just finished a specialist training programme in gynaecology but have decided that you would like to change your speciality to psychiatry. Would you go the library and get out the last three years of the Journal of Psychiatry, surf the net for the latest ideas, or go to a textbook to give the subject some form and coherence? You might well try all three though the latter would provide a map with the main features highlighted and routes to the important problems and solutions. Then you can go to the web and the journals with the key concepts in place and a balanced view of the topic.

The textbook is not dead (it can of course be electronic) but its function has become clearer. It provides a particular view of the organisation of knowledge provided by an individual writer (or group of writers). This must be the case or all textbooks would be the same. Hence the need and value of diversity. They are not, and could not, be the most up-to-date reference work. We now have better ways of doing this by electronic means. But they provide the map of a subject into which a wide range of knowledge and experience fills in the details. Textbooks provide the means of exploring a subject and providing the landmarks before going on the journey on your own. The great landmarks of the subject may change little with time but the detail is likely to be continually moving and changing, hence the need to supplement the text book with up-to-date information. Here then is a role for journals and the Internet.

THE INTERNET AND THE WEB. The power of computing and the ease, availability, and access to information have changed the way in which we can tell stories and get comments on them. "Lessons of the Week" can become lessons of the hour and a problem shared rapidly. The role of telemedicine and thus the visual display of information enhances this even more. Patients can tell their stories and others can listen and ask questions. Specialist web sites provide such a facility for doctors and those with a particular illness. Instead of sharing confidential patient information between doctors it becomes widely and publicly available. This has both great advantages and disadvantages.

The advantages are clear. Openness and clarity of information and methods of checking the story and the possible remedies are obvious. The support function for others with the same condition can be invaluable. Access to information and the answering of questions can provide great reassurance for all. The great power of the patient experience can be of enormous value and can be widely shared. In a more technical vein the ability to access the latest journals and scientific information can be for the benefit of everyone. To be able to check the doctor's story against those of others can be revealing. Patients can do this readily and bring their print-out to the surgery. And herein lies the disadvantage.

As the web expands, so does the range of information available, so some check will be required on its quality and validity. Who is giving information, and can it be verified and checked? This is not a defensive argument, in that only doctors of a particular seniority and accreditation can give proper advice. This is not the case. It is about trust and professional values. Patients need the reassurance that the information they obtain is reliable and broadly based. Patients need the whole story and not just part of it, edited, filtered and refined by a particular group. Increasingly, therefore, doctors and other health professionals are likely to be called on to interpret and review such information. They will need, therefore, to become familiar with the sources and be able to check them for themselves. This will require data searching and interpretative expertise to deal with this. Not for the first time in this book, the word exegesis is raised.

This leads naturally to a discussion of the use of large databases which give access to very large amounts of information based on the individual stories of thousands of people. They may be based on population studies or the collection of large amounts of clinical trial data. Whatever the source they are the ultimate check on the individual case. They are the benchmark of clinical and public health practice. No matter how interesting and unique an individual patient may be, it is essential to compare the story against current diagnostic thinking and management practice. They provide the evidence base for the individual. They are not mutually exclusive, or in competition. One is not right and the other wrong. Both methods need each other and feed on each other. Data banks alone miss the individuality of the person, and considering only the individual, misses the wealth of past and present experience world wide.

One of the best examples of bringing the two concepts together is in the writings of William Pickles, a general practitioner in Wensleydale. His book, "Epidemiology in a Country Practice" (W.N. Pickles, 1939, John Wright and Sons, Bristol) describes in detail the life and times of the people who live in a Yorkshire dale. He cares for them as individuals, but at the same time collects information on their illness in order to understand them better. He describes general practice as having a "unique opportunity" to do this kind of medical synthesis, bringing population and patient together.

MEDICAL STUDENTS IN LITERATURE. We are all students of medicine, and to that end we must never stop learning. But how are we, the medical students of the past, the present and the future described in the literature. This particular sub-set of literature and medicine has been chosen as it brings together the three themes of this book, learning, humour and storytelling. The student life is detailed less frequently in books and plays than that of the fully qualified doctor, or of illness and suffering. And yet the subject is interesting. Perhaps the most memorable comes from a brief glimpse of medical students in "Pickwick Papers" by Charles Dickens. The subject of the exchange is Bob Sawyer, the medical student.

"Nothing like dissecting to give one an appetite." Said Mr Bob Sawyer looking round the table.

Mr Pickwick slightly shuddered.

"By-the-by, Bob," said Mr Allen, "have you finished that leg yet?"

"Nearly", replied Sawyer, helping himself to half a fowl as he spoke. "It's very muscular for a child's."

"I've put my name down for an arm at our place," said Mr Allen. "We're clubbing for a subject, and the list is nearly full, only we can't get hold of any fellow that wants a head. I wish you'd take it."

"No," replied Bob Sawyer; "can't afford expensive luxuries."

"Nonsense!" said Allen.

"Can't indeed," rejoined Bob Sawyer. "I wouldn't mind a brain, but I couldn't stand a whole head."

It is a brilliant evocation of the nonchalance of the student, the bravado and the matter of fact nature of medical life. This tradition has been carried on in modern writers such as Richard Gordon in the "Doctor Books" (of which more later) and Colin Douglas, whose first novel, "A Houseman's Tale" (1975, Cannongate, Edinburgh) describes many of the experiences and pitfalls that we all went through.

Another rather unusual story in the same vein is called, "The Life History of a Medical Student. The Awful and Ethical Allegory of Deuteronomy Smith" . The author is anonymous, and it is set in Edinburgh, probably in the 1930s. Here is how the examinations are described.

"And it came to pass that at divers times Deuteronomy stood before the elders of the Temples of learning.

And the elders asked him many questions of the bones of men and of beasts, and concerning the herbs of the fields and the metals of the earth whereby the sicknesses of men are healed.

But lo! They were able to ask him nothing that he could not answer, and many wonderful deeds did he perform in their sight.

And because of these things, the elders of the Temple called upon Deuteronomy to appear again before them on a certain day.

And on that day, which was the first day of the eighth month of the year, Deuteronomy and many other young men stood in a great hall.

And they wore gowns adorned with hoods of many colours, and so bright were they that men said that Solomon in all his glory was not arrayed like one of these."

For someone who now sees many graduation days, this is a splendid reminder of its purpose, and pageantry.

But life is not all fun for the medical student. There are considerable stresses and strains and at times even boredom. In "Madame Bovary" by Gustav Flaubert, Charles, a medical student, records his feelings.

"The list of lectures which he read in the official timetable set his head in a whirl. They covered anatomy, pathology, physiology, pharmacy, chemistry, botany, clinical medicine and therapeutics, to say nothing of hygiene and materia medica-all words about the etymology of which he knew nothing, words which seemed to him like the portals of sanctuaries in which dwelt the shades of the august. He understood absolutely nothing. No matter how hard he listened, he made but heavy weather of the lectures. Nevertheless he worked, equipped himself with bound notebooks, attended all the courses, and never played truant. He accomplished his little daily task in the manner of a mill horse, which goes round and round in blinkers, doing what he does without knowing the reason for it."

Doesn't sound much fun. In Somerset Maugham's "Of Human Bondage" a similar picture is painted. Philip is a medical student and he comments on the conjoint examination, "He was eager to pass it since that ended the drudgery of the curriculum: after it was done the student became an out-patients' clerk and was brought into contact with men and women as well as with textbooks."

Thank goodness for problem based learning and the new curricula. Before that he discusses the difficulties and indeed the poverty associated with being a student, and it is not quite like Bob Sawyer's cheerful views of medicine. The difficulty of the examination process is again noted. Of those who have difficulties he comments:

"They remain year after year, objects of good-humoured scorn to younger men. Some of then crawl through the examination of the Apothecaries Hall: others become non-qualified assistants, a precarious position in which they are at the mercy of their employers: their lot is poverty, drunkenness, and heaven only knows their end. But for the most part medical students are industrious young men of the middle class with a sufficient allowance to live in a respectable fashion."

Students and young doctors also have to face difficult problems and may take time to adjust and learn. A short story by Arthur Conan Doyle entitled "His First Operation" shows how it might be done.

"It was the first day of the winter session, and the third year's man was walking with the first year's man. Twelve o'clock was just booming out from the Tron Church.
    "Let me see," said the third year's man, "you have never seen an operation?"
    "Never"
    "Then this way please. This is Rutherford's historic bar. A glass of sherry, please, for this gentleman. You are rather sensitive, are you not?"
    "My nerves are not very strong I'm afraid."

And so the story continues, with more sherry, a white face, and dreadful expectations. They arrive at the operating theatres where the conversation continues.

"There's going to be a crowd at Archer's," whispered the senior man with suppressed excitement." It's grand to see him at work. I've seen him jab all around the aorta until it made me jumpy to watch him."

Not perhaps the best preparation for your first operation. He faints of course at the first sight of the patient and wakens lying on the floor, and misses the critical part; the patient didn't stand the chloroform and the operation was cancelled. In a slighter lighter mode Richard Gordon in "Doctor in the House" describes the medical student's first delivery. The text is interesting but those who remember the film will realise just how touching it was. The scene is set as Simon Sparrow, medical student, arrives at the house.

"Her time is near, doctor," said grandma with satisfaction.

"You have no need to worry any longer, missus," I said brightly...

"Mother," I said earnestly, "How many children have you?"

"Five, Doctor", she groaned. Well that was something. At least one of us knew a bit about it....

"I think it's coming doctor!" she gasped, between pains. I grasped her hand vigorously...."I feel sick", she cried miserably. "So do I", I said. I wondered what on earth I was going to do....Out of my hip pocket I drew a small but valuable volume in a limp red cover," The Student's Friend in Obstetrical Difficulties." It was written by a hard-headed obstetrician on the staff of a Scottish hospital who was under no illusions about what students would find difficult. It started off with the "Normal Delivery"....I glanced at the first page, "Sterility" it said...The newspaper that was it.. and I scattered over the floor and the bed.

"Is it come yet" she (grandma) said. "Almost" I told her. "I shall need lots more water."

"It's coming, doctor!".....Suddenly I became aware of a new note in the mother's cry - a higher wailing muffled squeal. I dropped the soap and tore back the bedclothes....

"Do you do a lot of babies, doctor?" asked the mother. "Hundreds," I said, "Every day."

"What's your name doctor, if you don't mind?" she said. I told her. "I'll call 'im after you. I always call them after the doctor or nurse, according."

And the baby is thus called Simon.

In spite of all that is written about the bravado and callousness of the student they are capable of great compassion and sensitivity, as all who teach them know. They are a wonderful group and it is a privilege to teach them. This is perhaps best brought out in a story by Dr John Brown, an Edinburgh physician in the mid 19th century, at a time before the use of anaesthetics. The story is called "Rab and his Friends." Rab is the dog whose master, James, brings his wife to the Royal Infirmary with a breast lump. The medical students become involved in the care and Ailie, the patient, eventually goes to the operating theatre. The scene is set for the operation and is narrated by the medical student.

"The operating theatre is crowded; much talk and fun, and all the cordiality and stir of youth. The surgeon and his staff of assistants is there. In comes Ailie: one look at her quiets and abates the eager students. That beautiful old woman is too much for them; they sit down and are dumb and gaze at her. These rough boys feel the power of her presence. She walks in quickly, but without haste; dressed in her mutch, her neckerchief, her white dimity shortgown, her black bambazeen petticoat, showing her white worsted stockings and her carpet shoes. Behind her was James, with Rab. James sat down in the distance, and took that huge and noble head between his knees. Rab looked perplexed and dangerous; forever cocking his ear and dropping it fast.

Ailie stepped up on a seat, and laid herself on the table, as her friend the surgeon told her; arranged herself, gave a rapid look at James, shut her eyes, rested herself on me, and took my hand. The operation was at once begun: it was necessarily slow; and chloroform - one of God's best gifts to his suffering children - was then unknown. The surgeon did his work. The pale face showed its pain but was still and silent. Rab's soul was working within him; he saw that something strange was going on - blood flowing from his mistress, and she was suffering; his ragged ear was up, and importunate; he growled and gave now and then a sharp impatient yelp; he would have liked to have done something to that man. But James had him firm, and gave him a glower from time to time, and an imitation of a possible kick; - all the better for James, it kept his mind and his eye off Ailie.

It is over: she is dressed, steps gently and decently down from the table, looks for James; then, turning to the surgeon and students, she curtsies; - and in a low clear voice begs their pardon if she has behaved ill. The students - all of us - wept like children; the surgeon helped her up carefully - and, resting on James and me, Ailie went to her room, Rab following."

SOME CONCLUSIONS

Medical stories, from aphorisms to the Internet, are a fascinating way of learning medicine, and learning about the profession. Case histories, log books and textbooks have served the profession well over generations. The newer media from telemedicine to the Internet have much to add to the process of learning. Students now have a huge range of material available to stimulate and enthuse. Their curiosity can be tested and satisfied.

Being a medical student is a great privilege. This author still thinks of himself as one. Learning, laughing, dealing with disease and illness and finding out how best to care for people. Continuing to be a student throughout life is even more rewarding as it allows the transmission of experience and values from one generation to another, and to tell others what a wonderful profession it is. Even older students learn from younger ones and this maintains the continuity of professional values and aspirations.

7. Other Ways of Telling Stories

"Words! Pens are too light. Take a chisel to write." *Basil Bunting.*

It should not be assumed that all stories need to be told in a particular way, for example, orally or in written prose, methods we have concentrated on so far in this book. As the quotation from Basil Bunting at the start of this chapter makes clear there are many other ways in which messages can be delivered, emotions stirred, lessons learned, and tales told, without the use of language, in written or oral form. Body language, our natural way of responding to the world around us, is particularly powerful in this regard. In addition language can be used in the form of poetry, opera, songs, and even hymns to tell tales. This chapter thus looks at a range of alternative ways of telling stories, such as dance, music, mime and the visual arts. One particular art form which brings humour, storytelling and art together is cartoon drawing, and this will be described in detail later in this chapter.

1. **BODY LANGUAGE.** How our bodies respond to events clearly reflects on our innermost feelings. Fear, outrage, anxiety, concern, love, are all expressed in our faces and our body movements. We are seen to be defensive, welcoming, angry, caring by how we stand and how we move. We unconsciously tell stories and send messages using our body all the time, and some of us do this more obviously than others. Some of us wear our hearts on our sleeves. We do not need to say anything, it is visible for all to see. Other people watch us, and we watch them. We learn attitudes and how (and how not) to deal with people and respond to their concerns. Controlling such images can be difficult. Making such images neutral and non-judgmental may be necessary at times, in spite of our wish to respond.

There is a cartoon which depicts a general practitioner at the door of his (yes his) consulting room, looking into the surgery waiting room. He is wearing a tee shirt on which is printed the message, "Campaign for real ailments". It says it all. Don't bother me with trivia, I'm a doctor and I only see real illnesses. It's a wonderful image (it cannot really be true can it?), and one which provokes discussion and debate.

The senior clinician on a ward round rapidly conveys his or her feelings and attitudes about patients. The stories they tell by their non-verbal signals constitute the hidden agenda of clinical practice. Yet this comprises a substantial part of the unwritten curriculum by which medical students and others learn habits and attitudes. Its power cannot be ignored. These body postures (our body postures) may say more about our attitudes than words can about how we approach patients, listen to them, leave them, comfort them. In media appearances or in facing the public, the looks, openness, use of the hands and facial movements all send out signals about the problem being discussed, its seriousness and the concern of the person telling the story.

It is often useful to share with patients one's own feelings and attitudes. It builds a sense of trust and openness. But just as it is important to choose our words carefully so it is important not to overstate the case by our non verbal language. For example, on seeing a suppurating wound, one's first reaction may have been one of revulsion and fear. But it would not necessarily be appropriate to display this at first glance. Similarly, in breaking bad news the non verbal response must be appropriate. This is perhaps what Osler (1939) meant by "Aequanimitas", or equanimity. The ability to see and do things with an attitude which is comforting and does not over-react, no matter how one might wish to. The balance between involvement and disinterest is a difficult one to play out in practice. What is clear is that the stories we tell with our faces, hands and bodies are a central part of it.

Perhaps the lesson to learn is that what we do with our non verbal language matters to patients and the public at large. They watch us carefully and with great interest, and often in our most unguarded moments when we are tired and uncertain. Being a professional can be difficult, but it is what our patients expect.

2. **TOUCH.** This is very closely related to our non verbal body language. It is often said that it is possible to divide doctors into two classes, the "touchers" and the "non-touchers". Watching doctors on a ward round can be very revealing, as it says much about how they communicate with patients. Feeling the pulse can have several functions, one of which is to make connections with patients and allow them to realise that there is someone who is prepared to make that contact with them and help them.

As always sensitivity in this matter is crucial and the possibility of "touch" being misinterpreted is very real.

Some doctors seem to have the ability to make touch part of the therapy. The therapeutic benefit is real if inexplicable. The narrative conveying more than just contact, it is much more. To go as far as to say that healing occurs would perhaps be stretching the evidence. Still it is important to remember that touch is part of the doctor's repertoire, and used appropriately, and under supervision and with safeguards, it can tell the patient a great deal about them and you. In the film of the book "Patch Adams"(Adams and Mylander, 1998), the real story of an American doctor who believes in humour, mime and touch in the healing of patients, the main question posed for me was the effector mechanism of the technique. But perhaps we should not be too concerned about the physiological pathways of a technique which brings benefits to patients. We didn't know how insulin worked for many years.

3. **MIME AND CLOWNING.** Reference has already been made to the use of mime and clowning in telling stories to patients. There is an increasing use of such techniques in clinical practice, particularly in the paediatric setting. It allows feelings and anxieties to be explored and for children, in a situation which may appear to be unreal, touch reality. The addition of humour and laughter also has a therapeutic benefit and makes it easier to deal with difficult problems. To do this effectively requires full co-operation of the hospital and professionals involved, but those who have experience of it tell good stories of its value. Perhaps we should not be frightened to try new things just because they are different. The old Guinness advert comes to mind. "I don't like it because I haven't tried it".

4. **CLINICAL SKILLS AS NON VERBAL STORIES.** Some non verbal stories reflect the skills and attitudes of those doctors who have special gifts. They may be surgeons or physicians, but to watch them at work is a pleasure and an education. They simplify, as all good stories do, a complex and difficult task, and they can make the operation or procedure appear almost beautiful. There is an economy of effort and a rhythm which has been developed by practice and care. With delicacy and sensitivity the skilled surgeon performs something akin to a work of art. Restoring and healing. In a similar way a clinical examination or procedure performed with the weight of experience and wisdom tells a story

about the professionalism of the medical profession. We tell others about these skills and learn from them in the same way as we would if they were recounted in the classroom.

5. **STORIES AND THE ARTS.**   The arts, other than literature, have a remarkable ability to tell a story and to arouse emotions and feelings. Music, dance and the visual arts all provide an essential function in opening up new experiences and telling tales which are able to lift hearts and give rise to tears. Not everyone is moved by the same experience, and some respond more to music, others to dance, and others to painting or sculpture. They are all ways of communicating. Each of these will be considered in turn.

Music.   Music can provide a powerful way of telling stories, happy, sad, light, profound and solemn. When associated with words in song or opera that power can be increased considerably. Music can stir memories of other stories and events, and bring back recollections of places and people. Music from the popular culture of the 1960s or 1970s can bring back to a certain age group feelings of youth and experiences now no longer part of life. Music can be soothing or stirring and excite or annoy. The bagpipes, for example, stir mixed emotions. Music can have healing powers, and uplift and strengthen. A verse from a poem of a 17th century Scottish doctor John Armstrong (1709-79) entitled "The Art of Preserving Health" sums this up well.

> "Music exalts each joy, allays each grief,
> Expels diseases, softens every pain,
> Subdues the rage of poison, and the plague;
> And hence the wise of ancient days ador'd
> One power of physic, melody and song."

Even hymns tell a story, often a very powerful one (Watson, 1997). Titles such as "Tell me the old, old story" would be typical of this. A well known hymn such as "Once in Royal David's City" is a straight story in verse and put to music. There are many others however which reflect on the emotions and feelings around the major events in life. Later in this book we will discuss the "contagious theory of behaviour change". Hymns have been known to have that power, such is the effect of music and poetry combined with a message which is tailored to an individual.

The visual arts. Painting and sculpture can have a profound effect on people. The old adage that "every picture tells a story" is certainly true. The work of the artist can conjure up a vision which illuminates an event or an emotion. With sculpture this also becomes touchable and can achieve a closeness and an intimacy in a way which a painting may not. The size of the painting does not seem to matter in terms of the effect it produces. Art in hospital can be of value, and the appropriate choice of paintings in a ward, a room, or a reception area can be helpful. Indeed the whole area of design of a health service environment (building or external environment) is relevant.

An interesting exercise for everyone to do is to consider the way in which the artist begins to "compose" the picture. Starting with a subject, almost any subject, the artist has to decide in the same way as the author does, just what has to go onto the canvas, what are to be the highlights and the main features, and the overall impression the picture has to make. Take a topic such as the crucifixion and consider how different artists have painted this and given a different focus, atmosphere and dynamic to the painting. A visit to any art gallery will show how differently artists have painted portraits. Not just in style or colour, but of background and setting. They tell different stories. The use of symbols and allusions all add to the meaning of the picture. And it is this word "meaning" which connects the painting to the story.

Part of this discussion relates to the architecture and design of buildings, particularly health care settings such as hospitals or primary care facilities. Attention to detail in the design of such buildings is relevant and there is sufficient evidence that they make people feel better when looked after in appropriately designed buildings, that it tells stories about those who work in them and manage them. In addition there is a need to make people feel welcome in hospitals, and the design of the front entrance and how they are greeted is all part of this. Some health settings have very special functions, for example as a place of care for those with learning difficulties. In these the use of textures, surfaces and sounds, water, music and movement can all add to the therapeutic environment. Light colour, space and the quality of the furnishings all help. The use of plants, trees, and greenery can be of great value. They tell a story of the care taken in the planning of the health setting. This is not just about new developments, it's about re-thinking older buildings and using imagination and creativity to improve the ambience.

Sculpture. The use of sculpture in a hospital environment is another way of telling a story. This can be abstract, or represent a real person or event. It can be available to be touched or looked at. The statue at the entrance of the Liverpool maternity hospital depicts a healthy woman, safely delivered of her baby, and ready to breast feed it. The whole story is there. The process of delivery, the successful outcome and the health promotion exercise for the mother after delivery. A completely different example is the Gateshead Angel by Anthony Gormley. It is a wonderful piece, a huge figure with outstretched wings high above the A1 in the north of England. It excites pleasure, anger and many other emotions. But it is a symbol (a story) of regeneration and hope. It cheers many people up in the morning as they sit in the traffic, and infuriates others!

Dance. Movement and dance are fascinating ways of telling stories and conveying feelings and emotions. Ballet would be the high point of this though there are many other ways in which movement can be used. The therapeutic benefit of dance is also real and not as well known as it might be. Children's games are of course a variant of this in which there may be both competition and fun. Ring-a-ring-roses would be a good example of this, recording as it does a method of preventing, and then catching the plague. Country dancing and folk dances often also contain the essence of a long lost tale, and the symbolism of the dance may remind us of this.

Theatre, film and television. These newer media contain all the elements for the telling of tales. They can be remarkably powerful, though in each instance what is provided is a fixed view of a story and sometimes not the one written by the author. The producer and director edit and set the story in a particular mode and in a particular way. It is less possible to use one's own imagination to relive the story if this has already been done by someone else. It is often difficult to read the book having seen the film. Yet the power is unmistakable.

Television and the related and newer Internet media also provide a similar way of recording a performance. For some productions, particularly the "soaps" it is possible to incorporate messages and educational opportunities. The "Archers" on the radio is a programme which has been doing this for decades. So it is with "East Enders" where subjects such as mental health, HIV infection, and many others have been covered. There is a significant learning opportunity from such programmes.

The theatre is generally a more intimate medium, and it is possible to see productions of the classics, such as the plays of Shakespeare, being performed in different costumes, settings and time periods, all using the same words. These productions thus present a particular view of the play, and this, in a much less grandiose way, is similar to a health professional repeating (performing) to a medical audience the script written by the patient. It is our interpretation of the history.

So far it has been assumed that the arts are ways of telling stories and of setting out, using painting, music, theatre or film to make others think, or to amuse and entertain. They can also be viewed from the alternative perspective, and, just as creative writing might be therapeutic, so also can the individual's involvement in the arts. This too has benefits (Nuffield Trust 1999). These benefits are real, both in improving the quality of life and making us feel better. They are wonderful ways of relaxing, learning, and being creative. The work of Murray Cox (1992) in Broadmoor Prison using Shakespeare with those committed to life sentences, is a particularly powerful example.

6. **POETRY.** Poetry is a particular form of writing and storytelling and is perhaps so important that it deserves a section of its own. It may or may not use rhyme, and its function, according to Hugh McDiarmid is:

> "The function, as it seems to me,
> O' poetry is to bring to be
> At lang, lang last that unity...

It is the synthesis and the unity which makes poetry so interesting. Poems do many things, they amuse, they educate, and they tell stories in a wonderfully imaginative way. To illustrate some of the ways in which poetry can do all of these things, the themes of this monograph, a number of examples will be used. Inevitably they will chosen by the author of this book. This, of course, is part of the process of editing, and the choices reflect a particular and personal interest. One of the tasks of the reader is to find better and more interesting examples. If this section stimulates that exercise, it will have been worthwhile.

Poems, just like good prose, have a remarkable way of using language. Poets are able to concentrate language and send "shafts of light" into dark places. Some of the first lines of poems show how a few words, creatively and imaginatively put together, can provoke the most wonderful images and immediately engage the reader. Here are a few examples of opening lines, there are many more.

"Shall I compare thee to a summer's day?
Thou art more lovely and more temperate." *William Shakespeare*

"License my roving hands, and let them go
Before, behind, between, above , below.
O my America, my new found land,
My kingdom, safeliest when with one man mann'd." *John Donne.*

"Earth has not anything to show more fair.
Dull would he be of soul who could pass by
A site so touching in its majesty." *William Wordsworth.*

"Not a drum was heard, not a funeral note,
As his corpse to the rampart we hurried." *Charles Wolfe*

You want to read on and listen to more, and though all are different in tone and subject they hold you entranced. This seems so much better than,

"This is a 58 year old Caucasian male, who presented at the emergency department last night with right sided abdominal pain...."

But perhaps we can't use verse on all occasions!

Narrative poems are another important group. Their purpose is to tell a story and to do it in a way which engages and is memorable. This latter point is important as in past times children were invited to remember long sections of such poems. While in the concepts of modern learning this may be frowned on, those who went through the process can still remember the key verses some decades later. Such poems as "The Song of Hiawatha", "The Lay of the Last Minstrel", and "The Rime of the Ancient Mariner", and many others are wonderful stories in themselves, and are written in a way which invites you to read on. Take the three examples given, first "Hiawatha" by Henry Wadsworth Longfellow. This extract is from early in the poem and establishes Hiawatha's background.

"Ye who love the haunts of Nature,
Love the sunshine of the meadow,
Love the shadow of the forest
Love the wind among the branches
And the rain-shower and the snow-storm,
And the rushing of great rivers
Through their palisades of pine-trees.
And the thunder in the mountains
Whose innumerable echoes
Flap like eagles in their eyries:-
Listen to these wild traditions
To this song of Hiawatha."

The rhythm and the power of this engage you and make you want to read more
As an exercise, see how much better this is when read aloud, than silently.

Then to a few lines of Walter Scott's long poem, "The Lay of the Last Minstrel"

"Breathes there a man with soul so dead,
Who never to himself has said,
This is my own my native land"

And finally to "The Rime of the Ancient Mariner" by Samuel Taylor Coleridge.

"It is an ancient Mariner
And he stoppeth one of three.
By thy long beard and glittering eye
Now wherefore stopp'st thou me?"

Each of these poems, and you can read more in the Oxford book of Narrative
Verse, (Opie and Opie 1983) takes a major tale, turns it into poetry and makes
it both enjoyable and memorable. As an Annexe to this volume the
introductory section of Scott's narrative poem, "Harold the Dauntless" is
given as another example.

Reference has already been made to the way in which poems are remembered
and thus can be recalled when required. Rote learning is not fashionable, yet the

mechanism by which we remember, by which our memory is fashioned, is of great importance. How do we learn and remember was discussed in chapter 5.

Humour is another interesting facet of poetry. Humourous poems present a fascinating way of looking at a subject. There are a huge range, many of which have a medical theme. Here is only one example from William McGonnigle on the subject of drinking alcohol.

> "Oh, thou demon drink, thou fell destroyer;
> Thou curse of society and its greatest annoyer.
> What hast thou done to society, let me think?
> I answer thou hast caused the most of ills, thou demon drink."

Or take this description of syphilis from Alan Ramsey's Poem on Health (1684-1758)

> "Then, expect the terrible Attack
> Upon thy Head thy Conduit, Nose and Back;
> Pains through thy Shoulders, Arms, and Throat and Shins,
> Will threaten Death, and damn thee with thy sins.
> How frightful is the loss, and the disgrace
> When it destroys the beauties of the face!
> When the arch'd Nose in rotten ruin lies,
> And all the venom flames around the eyes;
> When the Uvula has got it's mortal wound
> The tongue and lips form words without a sound;
> When hair drops off, and Bones corrupt and bare
> Through ulcerated tags of muscle stare."

There are many more examples of poetry in a medical context, including a remarkable book by Zachary Cope on "The Acute Abdomen in Rhyme".

7. **CARTOONS AND CARICATURES.** Caricatures and cartoons represent a complete story in a single picture, a few lines on a page. They generally make you laugh, and, even though they may be of funny little men and women, contain animals who speak, or be of stylised buildings, plants and aliens, they seen real. The range of subjects for cartoons is almost infinite, and this section will

consider a specific sub-set, those with a broadly medical or health interest. To do this without the drawing in front of you is difficult and all the reader's imagination will be needed.

The earliest medically related caricatures tended to show doctors in a rather poor light. They were often depicted as trying, unsuccessfully, to conjure patients back from the dead, showing the impotence of medicine. The doctor was usually recognisable by the piss-pot, the symbol of scientific medicine. As an example of this rather negative perception one cartoon shows the doctor trying to take a foreign body from the eye of the patient while having an even larger mote in his own eye. There are an interesting series of 16th century cartoons of the physician, the surgeon and the apothecary, and the stereotypes are still recognisable. The surgeon is a man of action full of instruments of a cutting nature. The physician is quite different, he is wise and learned, slow and surrounded by books. He speaks wisdom at all times. The apothecary is a mixture of both, and carries the most appalling looking rectal syringe. You will agree that these characters still exist and it is interesting to consider that they are not new, but were recognised centuries ago.

The cartoons are also particularly good at describing diseases and illnesses. Gout is the classic with a crab, the claws of which are biting into the great toe. But others on colic, headache and ague are beautifully illustrated. Treatment given is even more fascinating. The older cartoons demonstrate the effect of the cowpox vaccination by showing a cow's heads growing from the recipient's arms and legs. By the beginning of the 20th century immunotherapy was just beginning and there is a cartoon which shows Von Behring (a most distinguished immunologist) at the pharmacist dispensing serum from a horse with the aid of a tap fixed to the animal's abdomen. The shape of things to come. Modern treatments are not immune from this treatment. There is a cartoon set in a gentleman's club with one of its senior members saying, "would you mind moving out of the light, I have a solar powered pacemaker".

Doctors, and their behaviour come out badly in the process, and over the centuries numerous cartoons have illustrated their weaknesses. They sometimes seem to be more interested at times in taking the fee and in their women patients than would seem appropriate. They are also chastised, and not so gently, for their clinical competence. In one cartoon there is a group of doctors examining a lady who has an obvious abdominal swelling. The first doctor says, "I think it's a collection of wind". The second, "I think it's a collection of water". The third, "I think it's a collection of wind and water", and the final doctor says, "I think if we just wait a few months she will deliver a baby". So much for diagnostic skills. Another well known 18th century cartoon shows the Faculty making an address to Mr Influenzae, thanking him for his kind visit to the country. They have made a great deal of money out of him and they invite him back. I doubt if many doctors after the 1999-2000 flu outbreak would feel the same. Doctors also appear very naive. There is a delightful 18th century French cartoon which shows a doctor examining a patient and, as if to show his competence, and boost patient confidence, he says, "I'm delighted, you have yellow fever, it's the first I have ever seen". The modern late 20th century equivalent is of the surgeon dancing in the ward, with the caption. It's the kind of operation he's always wanted to do". All this will, of course, change with the introduction of clinical governance.

Medical students are treated with the same disrespect. A cartoon of the first women medical students shows the profession reacting with horror, and a statue of Aesculapius in the background has his eyes closed unable to look. A particular favourite is of the medical student, examining a patient, and he asks the patient to put out his tongue. The caption reads, "Put out your tongue, and while it's out tell me what's wrong with you". This is the kind of gauche remark medical students are capable of. Another is the question asked by a medical student, as part of taking the history from a patient, "How long have you lived in poverty".

Patient views are also well represented in cartoons, and the procedures through which they are put. One cartoon depicts a patient being examined by a group of doctors with an endoscope in every orifice. A one-stop shop it might be, but it lacks a certain dignity. Public health issues are also of interest as they show the great sophistication of the public and their understanding of medical issues. For example, the cartoon of two farmers talking over a gate with bright sunshine overhead, saying to each other, "Turned out nasty again", illustrating their understanding of the connection between sunlight and skin cancer.

In each of the headings above there are many more examples which could be given.

But how do these cartoons relate to the theme of this book, bringing together stories, humour and learning? The humour is clear, as are the stories told by the cartoons. The learning process is similar to that described in chapter 4. Three points are relevant.

1. It is often easier to remember cartoons than text or oral presentations.

2. The basis of the learning is that the learner already knows something of the background of the humour (the learning example), and that he or she can connect with it. For example there is a good cartoon whose caption is "How do you feel after your vasectomy?" To which the reply is "It's made a vas deferens". It is impossible to understand this if you don't know what the vas is. Hence the fundamental principle, "The most important thing about learning is what the learner already knows".

3. The cartoon generally brings together in one picture two contradictory ideas, which spark off each other and create a new idea. And this is what happens in some forms of learning, namely that there is a shifting of concepts and ideas which results in something new and different being perceived. This then results in a change of behaviour.

Cartoons can specifically be used in a learning environment to act as trigger points for discussion and debate. For example there is a cartoon which shows a doctor's surgery with his name on it and his qualifications. They are as follows. "Dr Jones. MD, FRCS. HIV." This is the kind of cartoon which can be used to stimulate a discussion on attitudes to those who are HIV positive, and specifically when it is a doctor or another health care worker. A second example would be the cartoon which shows the doctor as a bull fighter, with the patient lying down totally submissive and pricked by needles and instruments. The doctor has total dominance. While this is only a caricature it does raise issues of control and autonomy. As a final example there is a cartoon which shows a small aeroplane flying across the Australian outback. The plane is called "The Flying Receptionist", and the caption reads "You can't get near the bloody doctor these days". Such a cartoon would raise issues of accessibility, friendliness and patient satisfaction. Once again many more examples could have been used to illustrate the learning potential of cartoons.

It is hoped that sufficient has been said to strengthen the claim that cartoons are not only funny, and tell a good story, but that they have high educational value. They can also have a real place in the teaching of medicine and in related professional groups, including managers and non-executive members of Trusts and Boards.

CONCLUSIONS

These brief remarks illustrate the importance and value of other ways of telling stories. There is a very rich diversity and those who teach facilitated learning may wish to use the range more fully. They are powerful and can change attitudes and feelings. We need to recognise their relevance and to pay as much care and attention to them as we do to other types of stories.

REFERENCES

Adams,P, and Mylander,M. Gesundheit! 1998. Healing Arts Press, Rochester, Vermont.

Cope, Z. The Acute Abdomen in Rhyme. 1962. H.K.Lewis, London.

Cox, M. Shakespeare Come to Broadmoor. The Actors Come Hither. The performance of tragedy in a secure psychiatric hospital. 1992. Jessica Kingsley, London.

The Nuffield Trust. Humanities in Medicine. Beyond the Millennium.1999.

Opie, I and Opie, P. The Oxford Book of Narrative Verse. 1983, Oxford University Press.

Osler, W. Aequinimitas: With other addresses to medical students, nurses and practitioners of medicine. 3rd Edition, 1939, H.K.Lewis, London.

Watson. J.R The English Hymn. A critical and historical study. 1997. Clarendon Press, Oxford.

8. Stories and Ethics

"Read not to contradict and confute, nor to believe and take for granted, nor to find talk or discourse, but to weigh and consider." *Francis Bacon in "On Studies".*

This chapter considers another dimension in the relationship between stories and learning, that of ethics. It is divided into three related parts. The first deals with stories themselves and how they influence our values. The second section considers how we learn and teach ethics, and how tales and legends can modify our beliefs. The final section opens up the question of changing values, evolutionary ethics, and how our beliefs may change. There is a considerable literature on this subject some of which will be reviewed in this chapter (Coles, 1989, Nelson,1997, Murray,1997, Greenhalgh and Hurwitz, 1998, Zeldin, 1998).

Stories and Ethics. Stories present us with interesting ways of seeing the world and reflect the views of others on substantial aspects of life and values. Most stories have within them some form of moral either in an overt way, or buried deep in the story itself. "Goodies" and 'baddies" are at the heart of many stories. Some clearly set out to support a particular view of the world, and parables would be the most obvious examples of this. But the sagas, fables, and stories and tales of heroes and legends are all underpinned by a set of values that support the culture and sustainability of the group itself. They are therefore an important way of learning about the world and how to behave.

In a more subtle way children's stories do exactly the same. They outline what is important and how one might behave. Those stories based in a school setting would be good examples of this. They set values of language and behaviour; in school, on the sporting field and in excitement and adventure. Both boys and girls are part of this, and with girls in particular they set out what is proper and what is not. They establish the culture into which a child might enter and create an often unobtainable world for some children, but one to which they might aspire. The hidden agenda is often very close to the surface. The holiday reading chapter in this book (Annexe 1) sets out some of these stories and they illustrate the power which they had, and in some instances still have. The political correctness of many such stories has been questioned in recent years.

More serious stories have done much to change the thinking of society by pointing out the shortcomings and failures of the world in which we live. The work of the great public health pioneers such as Sir Edwin Chadwick, Sir John Simon and William Farr, who published on the real life examples, were reflected in the stories of the great Victorian authors of whom Charles Dickens would be the most obvious example. The poverty, illness and social deprivation are highlighted in a different way than in case studies and reports. "Sybil", a novel by Benjamin Disraeli, a 19th century British Prime Minister, opens up similar questions of poverty and exclusion. "Uncle Tom's Cabin" by Harriet Beacher Stowe would be another example of a book with a particular mission and ethical stance, aimed at abolishing slavery in the Americas.

Perhaps the clearest examples of the tension between good and evil come from two novels from Scottish authors. The first is by Robert Louis Stevenson (1850-1894), "The Strange Case of Dr Jekyll and Mr Hyde". It is the story of an upright and middle aged man who has always struggled with the concept of good and evil. He happens to concoct a potion which allows him to break his personality into two, and to change and become evil. He enjoys this but is able to reverse the process. However, as he continues to experiment he finds it more enjoyable to be evil until he cannot reverse the process, and evil triumphs. He retains enough goodness at the end to write his story down and explain the problem and then to commit suicide. The second book, "The Private Memoirs and Confessions of a Justified Sinner" by James Hogg (1770-1835) is even more disturbing. It concerns a young man who considers himself to be one of the "elect". Guided by another young man who cannot be seen by anyone else, he commits acts of appalling depravity. The evil wins. In the end he also commits suicide. Both of these books show the power of evil and how it can sometimes triumph.

One can therefore come to a general conclusion that stories can affect behaviour, and that the purpose of some stories is to do just that; to set standards, values and a moral base. The remainder of this chapter will be to look at some examples in more detail and to consider how stories can be used in the teaching of ethics.

Parables and moral stories. In some ways parables are amongst the easiest of stories to consider in this way. They set out to have a moral purpose but use the narrative approach to illustrate the issue. The approach itself is interesting. When asked "Who is my neighbour?" Jesus does not reply with a list of categories, or of groups that might fit. He responds with a story, that of the Good Samaritan, from which the reader has then to draw his or her own conclusions. When asked about abilities He tells the parable of the talents. In a similar way the parables of the seed falling on stony or fertile ground, or how to build a house on sand or rock have stood the test of time. By use of a narrative a particular point is made both powerfully and understandably. The illustrations fit the proposed message and show how the selection of an example to highlight a point can open up a new vista and create a different vision.

In addition to biblical parables other stories, both long and short, act in the same way. The fables and sagas would be very good examples of this. Their power is that they engage the reader in the story, while at the same time open up the moral agenda.

A very considerable part of this is the use of heroes in stories. They become role models for us all. James Bond, Luke Skywalker, Dickson McCunn (in John Buchan's novels), Dr Zhivago, Sherlock Holmes, Miss Marple, Becky Sharp in "Vanity Fair", Dorothea in "Middlemarch", Isabella in "Portrait of a Lady", Elizabeth Bennett in "Pride and Prejudice", and many others, give us people to look up to. "The Lord of the Rings" by Tolkien provides another example of a hero, Frodo, who conquers all difficulties to find the ring. It is difficult not to identify with such characters. The reader can guess at the author's preferences. It is an interesting after dinner conversation to discuss who would be your heroes and heroines from the published literature.

In some instances it is not the characters themselves but the setting of the story which tells the tale. In two modern novels, "Trainspotting" by Irving Welsh, and "The Woman who Walked into Doors" by Roddy Doyle it is the setting and the situation which is as memorable as the characters. In the first there is a remarkable description of modern culture, which includes alcohol, drugs and HIV infection, within which the reader can both identify problems and solutions, but also make up his or her mind as to where they see themselves. The second is about domestic violence which again sets the scene and identifies some of the problems. Neither is explicit about values, but the reader is left to make the choices from the very powerful stories which are told.

As a final example, pantomime brings together laughter, the absurd, pathos, full audience involvement, and a very strong moral view. The evil and the good in one story, and the goodies always win. "Peter Pan and the Lost Boys" would be perhaps the best example of this, in which the audience can even participate in the resuscitation of Tinkerbell. The power of good made visible and tangible. We want Tinkerbell to get better, and she must get better, but only if we help.

But there are downsides. First, there is an assumption that all of the values set out in the story are for good and clearly this is not necessarily the case, as illustrated above. Evil can also be portrayed and the "baddies" can be just as attractive as the "goodies". There is no way in which the idea of "goodness" can be presumed. Stories don't always have a happy ending, a clear moral, and be a force for "good". Indeed it would be a pity if they were.

The second downside is that values can and do change and what is "right" for one generation may not be for another. Values, attitudes and behaviour all change with time. Such evolutionary ethical principles are not as infrequent as might at first seem, and this is discussed in more detail in the final section of this chapter.

The third problem is that such values often fit into a particular culture in a particular geographical location. In a world which is international and "global", and in which multi-cultural aspects are important, individual stories representing one set of values may be of very limited appeal, and indeed may be offensive to others. Differences in culture and attitudes affect all of our lives, and of course the stories from other cultures add colour and excitement to our lives. However they can be confusing, ill understood and unhelpful at times. But these differences in values, as we shall see when we consider the teaching of ethics, are important in that such stories can be used to challenge our assumptions and to help us to think through our own values.

Epiphany and ethics. This form of thinking, the epiphanic dimension to ethical discussion, is well described by Hawkins (1997). It is a way of knowing which emphasises insights into ethical problems. In one sense it is a sudden flash of inspiration and clarity. We "see" what was hidden. In her article Hawkins gives some clinical examples of doctors, who after wrestling with a clinical problem for some time, "see" the right course of action. This method of knowing fits well into the three themes of this book, storytelling, humour and learning. All are associated with a creative wish, to discover or identify something new or different. It is the second way of knowing, the first being the rational logical and factual approach. This is different and is based on feelings and an inner and personal view. It is just as legitimate.

Literature and ethics. The previous section dealt with stories which set out specifically to have a moral reference point and the advantages and disadvantages of this approach have been considered. This section takes a wider perspective and considers the role of what might be called the "serious" literature in the setting of values. The most obvious examples are in the great novels and plays. They provide a backdrop against which the whole range of human emotions and feelings are exposed and though classical in nature this does not mean that they are not funny and amusing. The Shakespearean plays such as "Hamlet" and "Anthony and Cleopatra" deal with power and corruption. "King Lear" with the problem of ageing and family disagreements, and "Romeo and Juliet" with love and passion. They can be read and performed and appreciated at so many different levels. The moral issues they contain can be identified and debated.

Other authors do the same. Henrik Ibsen in "The Doll's House" explores the role of women in society and how to deal with a dominant male. In another of his plays, "The Enemy of the People" he considers the possibility of a public health cover up in a small Norwegian spa town. The politics and the local views conflict with the views of the local doctor and he has to make a stand for the good of the community. As the doctor who holds such views he is tormented and abused and has stones thrown at him. It is he who is seen as the enemy of the people. In response he speaks one of the great lines in public health.

"You should never have your best trousers on when you turn out to fight for freedom and the truth."

Many novels explore the problems of madness and mental health. It is often the setting, as in "Jane Eyre", which is the issue. But just as importantly the novels of Tolstoy, Dickens, Scott, Elliot and scores of others ask questions about the world and how we feel about it. It is for this reason that almost any book can be used to consider ethical issues, which raises the next issue in this chapter, that of teaching medical ethics. Before doing so, however, there is one related point which should be considered, that of a reading list for medical students. Sir William Osler set one out for the students at the beginning of the 20th Century, and Richard Verney who edited an edition of Olser's works called "The Student Life" in the 1950s produced an updated version. Our own work in the 1980s (Calman et al 1988) produced a further version and these are appended at the end of this chapter. The question for you, dear reader, is to suggest a book list for the medical student or health professional at the start of the 21st century.

Teaching ethics. Before looking at the role of narrative in the teaching of medical ethics it is perhaps worth considering why we need to teach ethics and values at all and indeed if it can be done. We need to ask what the purpose of such teaching might be. In addition it should be clear that it is the learning process which is most relevant rather than the teaching and thus the question as to what the added value of teaching might be needs to be raised and answered. The assumption is made in this discussion that values can be influenced and changed, and as a consequence behaviour altered and hence teaching has a purpose. This is a questionable assumption. The notion that a one-week course on medical ethics will change attitudes and behaviour seems at first sight to be far fetched, as indeed it is likely to be. The first point to be made therefore is that the teaching of ethics, and of values, is not a short-term exercise and just a box to be ticked off. It has to be part of the culture of the medical school and of the teaching and learning throughout the course (Downie and Macnaughton,1999).

So what then is the purpose of teaching ethics, and why might it be necessary? This is not a new question and whether virtue can be taught was discussed generations ago by Plato and others. It is probably true to say that by the time an individual reaches a university many of their attitudes will already be set. It will be upon those values that others of a particularly medical nature will have to be viewed. In any group of students it is likely that there will be many views, some held with great conviction, others with less. The range of materials which can enhance learning is wide and varied and covers books and articles on ethics and philosophy and related subjects, case histories, patient and public views, books, poems and stories which address particular ethical topics, either overtly or in a more hidden manner. Just as relevant, however, will be the informal learning from friends, family, teachers and other role models. So what then is the purpose of teaching ethics?

Each individual needs a framework within which one's own views can be placed. Such a framework provides a knowledge base and a language within which to discuss moral issues. It provides a philosophical background to ethical thinking and for medical issues it is supplemented by the medical and scientific knowledge of the student within which to understand the ethical issue. For example, in the area of fertility treatment, genetics, and cloning it gives an essential knowledge base from which to consider the ethical implications. This would be the traditional approach to ethics teaching and would provide the basis for the active consideration of contemporary moral issues. All of the methods described above might be used for this purpose. But it should be more than this and before considering the ways in which the use of stories might have a place here are some of the other issues raised in teaching in the teaching of ethics.

1. It should not be about expressing a particular view of the world unless this is explicit and can be disagreed with without prejudice.

2. It should help individuals to be clearer about their own views on ethical issues and why they believe and value what they do.

3. A broad view of ethical issues should help to understand the views of others who do not hold such beliefs, and where their values are derived from.

4. It should enable the person to be able to respond to those whose who hold different views.

The use of stories, and the arts generally, can be of value in several different ways.

The first of these uses patient stories and patient experiences. These, as always, can be very powerful and can illustrate so many ethical issues. As has been said elsewhere in this book listening to patients and to their feelings and concerns can be of enormous benefit. They place the theoretical textbook problem into the context of a real one. They give life and vitality and indeed meaning to the practice of medicine.

It would be wrong to assume, however, that patient stories will give an answer to a particular moral problem. At best they will give an answer to a particular problem and at worst will leave all of the questions unanswered. They can often do no more (and that is of course a great deal) than to raise issues in a way which allows discussion and debate to occur.

For the doctor such patient stories are not theoretical exercises. They are real and are likely to need to be tackled at some point in the course of a clinical career. Thus the opportunity as a medical student to have a dry run, as it were, can be of great value. Case conferences which discuss ethical issues often expose differences of opinion and this in itself can be valuable. To recognise that others may think differently to you can come as a shock. It also, therefore, provides the place, in a closed setting, for such differences of view to be exposed and discussed. What if you then still disagree with the conclusion? How would you react if this was a real situation? Therein lies the value of the patient experience in teaching.

From the public health point of view a similar function can be obtained from newspaper articles, letters to the editor, and television broadcasts which provide a wide range of opinions which can be debated and discussed. Newspaper cuttings provide a ready source of material with their stories of right and wrong for the teaching of medical ethics.

It is from such personal stories that it becomes possible to look at the wider background literature in ethics, philosophy, anthropology and medicine. These can be used as sources of reference, for guidance and to enhance the understanding of the topic. As has been stated in several other parts of this book patient stories alone are not sufficient, the literature needs to be consulted.

The second set of stories are those in books, poems, plays and short stories which can be used to stimulate discussion and debate. Some examples have already been raised in previous sections. The possibilities are limitless and have been written up in many places (See Calman et al 1988, Calman, 1997.) They provide another way of looking at a problem, of thinking through a difficult issue and seeing how others view an ethical dilemma. The evaluation of courses to teach such issues using literature is positive but much more work needs to be done.
The third way in which stories can help is through film and video. Some of the

most powerful stories have been presented in these media, and they cannot be discounted as teaching resources. Films such as Star Wars, Indiana Jones, True Grit at the one end and Good Bye Mr Chips, Citizen Kane, High Noon and Patton, and many others at the other end, are fascinating comments on society and its values. In a slightly trivial way the advertisements on radio and television do a considerable amount to change behaviour and encourage us to buy products or behave differently. They are one minute sound bites that tell stories in a particularly effective way. We could learn much from the skill and expertise which goes into the construction of such adverts, some of which are very memorable. As a final game for next year's Christmas party list the adverts you remember well and how they made you do something differently.

The problem of uncertainty. Many of the ethical issues which arise in clinical and public health practice are because of the uncertainty surrounding the outcome. While we can give probabilities for the outcome of many forms of treatment, or the average prognosis in a particular condition, it is much more difficult to be specific for the individual. Thus some of the problems of patient choice in clinical practice relate to not knowing exactly what the outcome might be. On a one-to-one level between the patient and the doctor this can be discussed and debated, experiences shared and a common action plan drawn up with the patient's full involvement. In public health terms this is a much more difficult task. It is technically not possible at present to discuss issues with 50 million people. Even if it were possible, and technically this could be achieved now, there is likely to be a wide range of opinion on the "correct" action to take. Here even the use of stories may have limitations. Uncertainty remains at the centre of problems of communication with patients and the public.

Evolutionary ethics, can values change?

There is a fascination about the nature of values and whether or not they can change. This section of the chapter is an examination of the proposition that values might change and thus have consequences for the way in which medicine is practised. Although the particular interests of this volume are in clinical practice, the question is also a general one.

The topic is also not a new one and T.H.Huxley gave the Romanes Lecture in 1893 on "Evolution and Ethics" which, while not dealing directly with the issue of the evolution of ethics, does make some important related points perhaps best described in the Prolegmena to the essay (Huxley, 1893). The first of these is that values have changed over time from primitive societies to the present. The second is that the mechanism of these changes is not genetic but is modified by a different process. The third is that the process of social ethics indeed acts in the opposite direction to the cosmic process (i.e. evolution) in that medical science and the wish to help others inhibits the process of survival of the fittest. Thus doctors can be seen as the main agents for interfering with nature. It is these social factors which are often transmitted by way of stories.

But first, two quotations. The first is from John Locke in his "Essay Concerning Human Understanding" Book 1, Chapter IV, paragraph 24,

"When men have found some general propositions that could not be doubted of, as soon as understood, it was, I know, a short and easy way to conclude them innate. This being once received it eased the lazy from the pains of search, and stopped the inquiry of the doubtful, concerning all that was once styled innate: and it was of no small advantage to those who affected to be masters and teachers, to make this the principle of principles, that principles must not be questioned."

The second comes from "Captain Correlli's Mandolin" by Louis de Bernieres.
"It's a question of science," said Weber "you cannot alter a scientific fact."
"I don't care about science. It's an irrelevance. It's a moral principle you cannot alter, not a scientific fact."

"We disagree."said Weber amiably "It's obvious to me that ethics change with the times as science does. Ethics have changed because of the theories of Darwin."

These two quotations set out the territory and the possible conflicts. Can values change, and if they do, what changes them? In brief, the conclusion is that values can and do change though certain core values may be unaltered over a long period of time. The changes which occur, particularly in medical terms, relate to changes in knowledge, changes in social and cultural values and norms and an individual's personal experience of life, which again may change over time. The mechanism of these changes will also be considered.

BUT TO BEGIN AT THE BEGINNING. For the last 25 years the author has had an interest in palliative care. In the early 1970s he was involved in a remarkable "think tank" with Dame Cicely Saunders during which we explored a range of aspects of what was then called terminal care. Over the years as he has watched this subject, first as a practitioner and latterly as an educationalist and civil servant, and now as a Vice-Chancellor, it has been evident that attitudes and values have changed. Here are three brief examples.

1. Communication and involvement with patients. In the 1960s and 70s communication with patients seemed to have a low priority, though one's own teachers were particularly skilled in the process. Patients were rarely told the diagnosis, and indeed what the patient was told was not conveyed to other doctors. In 1974 100 letters sent to general practitioners from a well-known surgical unit were reviewed. All patients had had the diagnosis of cancer confirmed. In all instances the GPs were told the diagnosis, the details of the surgical procedure including the type of sutures used, but in only two cases was the doctor told what the patient had been told about the illness. Again in 1974, when the author became a professor of oncology, it was very unusual for the patient to have been told of the diagnosis before referral. Things have now changed dramatically and for the better. Patients are seen as full partners in the process and informed and involved in decision making.

   Looking back to the student experience it is not difficult to see why such attitudes occurred. An extract from a Handbook of Clinical Methods widely used at the time, reproduced in chapter 3 of this book, says it all.

2. The concept of extra ordinary means. This concept which, in summary, says that in life saving decisions at the end of life only ordinary means should be used, that is, techniques which would be considered routine and not out of the ordinary. It is clear that over the years the definition as to what is ordinary and what is not ordinary has changed considerably and thus the decisions to be taken, and how far one can go to prolong life, become more difficult. If few methods are available the decisions become much easier than if a wide range of methods is available.

   In a similar way it is perversely much easier to make decisions about treating an illness if the illness cannot be treated, though not for the patient it should be added. Once treatment becomes available a whole range of new questions arise, from access to care, the costs of treatment, the facilities available and the choice of the patient. What a nuisance!

3. Euthanasia. It is also clear that public and professional views on euthanasia have changed over the years. The debate is more widespread and recent well-publicised cases both in the UK and overseas have stimulated this discussion. Those who 20 years ago might have dismissed the concept out of hand are now prepared to at least discuss the topic. Why has this happened? Part of the explanation must be that we are living longer and thus subject to an increasing number of debilitating diseases at a time when family structures are dissolving. Faced with this situation it is perhaps not surprising that some express the wish "not to be a burden". Such changes in social and cultural values are likely to impact on professional practice at some point and illustrates an issue which will be picked up later, namely that doctors and other health professionals are part of civil society and react to changes within it. We hear and listen to what others say. Their stories matter and we learn from them.

These three examples led us to look at other areas where changes in practice have resulted from changes in ethical principles. To begin with take the Hippocratic Oath and ask how many of the principles remain intact. Here are a few comments.

The Hippocratic Oath. Written in 4th century Greece the context and the content are quite different from today. There is no mention of rationing, public health or research. Still some important points emerge. Let's look at three.

1. Abortion. The Hippocratic Oath makes it clear that abortion should not be performed. Yet at the present time over one hundred thousand are carried out each year in this country by doctors, some of whom at least have taken the Hippocratic Oath.

2. Confidentiality. The Oath makes it clear that everything in the consultation should be kept secret and be confidential between the patient and the doctor. This is clearly not the case nowadays. Information is shared widely amongst the team and indeed circulated to a range of non-professionals for a variety of purposes.

3. For the benefit of patients. The Oath strongly suggests that the doctor's task is to do everything possible for the benefit of patients. Most doctors would agree with this but most would also recognise that this is just not possible in all circumstances. Resources and facilities may not be available for the best to be done.

These examples do not make the modern doctor less "virtuous", rather they illustrate the changes which have occurred.

Some further examples. Further examples can be used to illustrate the point that values have changed.

1. Health care reforms. Who would have believed 20 years ago that doctors in this country would be talking the language of the market. Cost benefit analysis, audit, priorities, rationing, governance, etc. all trip off the tongue with ease. What a remarkable change in values.

2. Lifestyle issues. Now that there is clear evidence that some lifestyle issues are closely associated with ill health, smoking being the obvious example, it was only a small step to suggest that those with smoking related illness should not be treated in the NHS as they had brought the disease on themselves. Such a view would not have been considered 20 years ago. Similarly with HIV infection, gross obesity and drug misuse.

3. Vaccination. Of all the techniques for improving health then vaccination is one of the most successful and cost effective. It is well recognised that there are a small number of complications known to result from the procedure. As the knowledge of the wild type infection recedes in the population there is a questioning as to whether or not they are needed. The disease has gone, hence the need for vaccination has disappeared. Again a very considerable change in views.

4. HIV infection. Initially HIV infection was seen as something related to gays, and not to "ordinary" people. Apart from some important players, including some very distinguished Chief Medical Officers, it was not taken very seriously. As a problem it had little consequence for the population. That began to change as the epidemic developed and the

heterosexual spread was recognised. The result has been a significant shift in behaviour, namely in the practice of "safe sex".

Changing values. If we accept for the moment that values can and do change (and many other examples could be used) what is it that causes the change? Three possible mechanisms can be considered.

Changes in the knowledge base. This is the most obvious and comes in two forms. The first is new knowledge about existing problems or techniques and the second from completely new areas of work. In the first category new drug treatments and modifications of existing surgical practice may all add to the ethical implications. However, it is in the brand new areas where completely original problems are created that most of the interest lies. Here are some examples.

1. Transplantation, including xenotranplantation. This was a very significant development. First with kidneys, and then hearts, lungs and livers. It meant that doctors had to re-think who owned an organ and who could give permission for it to be used. Xenotransplantation was even more interesting. But how was it different from the use of other tissues of animal origin in surgical practice?

2. Contraception, including emergency contraception. While contraception had always been available (usually from the hairdresser's shop under the counter) the advent of the contraceptive pill changed everything. It was readily available and easy to use. Coming as it did with a liberalisation of sexual attitudes it changed habits and behaviour. While things changed again with HIV infection and the need to use condoms, the process had begun. A new twist arose with the introduction of emergency contraception, the "morning after pill". It would now be possible to have casual sex and deal with the consequences the next day. How would doctors react? Was this not just like an abortion? Who would you have to tell, whose permission would need to be sought? What if the person was underage? None of these questions was new but the technology forced doctors and others to question again the basic values and beliefs and how they impinged on clinical practice.

3. Infertility treatment. This has developed very rapidly over the last 20 years. From artificial insemination to egg donation and surrogate mothers. Was it a disease anyway, and why should it be treated on the NHS? These and many other questions needed to be reviewed again.

4. Cloning and stem cell procedures. This is one of the most significant technical achievements in recent science. The possibilities are considerable but at the same time they raise major ethical issues. Should human cloning be allowed? How far should research be encouraged and funded? If it's not done in this country will others go ahead anyway? The fundamental questions of course relate to the concept of person-hood and how that might change if human cloning became a reality.

5. Genetic screening. This is not a new concept as the cruder process of family history taking has been used for decades. However, it is the sophistication of the technology and its broadening scope which has changed the picture. At the moment it is single gene defects which are the commonest of the genetic problems detected. In the future it will be complex patterns of genetic coding which will change the probability for the appearance of a disease. These raise important issues such as confidentiality of the information, employment prospects and insurance implications.

In the list given above a wide range of possibilities exists for significant change in how we think. If any of the implications and consequences come about then there will need to be a significant re-look at our values and concepts of ethical issues. In essence new knowledge indicates what we can and could do. The question which is raised is whether we ought and should do it.

It would be fair to say that perhaps with one or two exceptions there are no new ethical problems, only modifications of existing ones. Nevertheless they will alter our thinking. One new one is the principle of equal weight in which, contrary to previous practice where the wishes of the patient are paramount, the possibility arises that relatives of someone with a genetic disorder might have the right to know this information for their own benefit. This could mean telling a third party against the wishes of the patient. A second is the topic of cloning which, if it was applied to humans, could radically alter our thinking and practice.

Social values and attitudes. The first topic was about the science base and how knowledge could change behaviour. The second is about social attitudes and how we learn from others, the role of communication and listening. These have changed very considerably over the years and continue to do so. They are reflected in how we dress, how we use our increasing leisure time, how we view authority, and many others. Part of this process has been our changing views of major social and ethical issues. Examples of this might include:

1. Public views of the medical profession. There is now, quite properly, greater questioning of the role of doctors and the way in which the medical profession operates and regulates itself.

2. Less credence given to the role of the church and other sources of authority.

3. Increasing interest in human rights and now animal rights. The human rights movement has been growing and there is greater awareness as to what these rights are and how they can be used.

4. Religious intolerance and racial hatred. In spite of greater internationalisation, racial and religious intolerance is a major source of conflict across the world. It can be a significant barrier to change.

5. Rise in single issue groups, e.g., environment, health issues. Almost all illnesses and diseases have pressure groups whose function is, again quite properly, to fight for the rights of their own members. This can sometimes change the decision making process in a way which disadvantages other groups and in particular those patient groups who are less able to get organised and put their case.

6. Role of IT and the Internet. The ready access to information will also be a significant source of change. Patients already come to the clinic with their print outs, and this is likely to increase. The quality of information is likely to be a major problem. However as a vehicle for changing the medical profession it is likely to be very powerful.

7. Changing attitudes to the family and to sexual relations. Over the last 30

years we have seen very significant shifts in family life and attitudes to sex. Doctors, as part of society, cannot fail to be influenced by this, they are part of it. Contraception, abortion, the care of the elderly all fall into this category.

Even within a single population, of relatively small size, there will be significant variation in social and cultural views. This makes it particularly difficult to reflect all the views of society when a major decision has to be made, for example, on a risk issue. How this heterogeneity is expressed following a decision is sometimes difficult to predict. Suffice it to say that attitudes and values in society as a whole are constantly changing and the values within the medical profession reflect this. These social attitudes can be readily influenced and changed.

Personal experience gained over time. This is the third method of initiating a change in values and is clearly related to the first two mechanisms. There is little doubt that we all change with time. Our tastes, hobbies, political views and friendships all change. These are a result of experiences, some good and some bad. We learn through stories and real events what matters to us and what does not and this is the substance of this book. The personal nature of these experiences is important and can affect each of us profoundly and can cause us to completely change our minds.

There are therefore many ways in which our views, and those of society can change, and the medical implications of this are part of a more universal phenomenon. Doctors and their patients are part of society and would be expected to change in a similar way. This raises the question as to whether any values are fixed, social or professional, and this is a subject to be discussed shortly. But first a short digression to look at where values come from.

The source of our values. Our values are determined in a variety of ways, which include,

1. Social. We have already shown how rapidly values can change in whole populations.

2. Educational. Influences during the whole educational process, from school to continuing education, can be profound. Role models in particular can readily shape our views.

3. Family. Our family values are also important. We learn traits and mannerisms as well as attitudes and beliefs. These range from political and religious matter to football team support and hobbies.

4. Peers. In all walks of life whom we work with and look up to is important. We need heroes and legends to make life meaningful and in some instances give it purpose.

5. Professional. The process of professional education and recognition is a powerful source of attitudes and values. The hidden agenda is strong and it is generally necessary to conform. Those who do not can sometimes find it difficult. Tribalism and group feelings are important, as is a specific culture which can only be understood from the inside. Elsewhere in this book it has been suggested that all professional speciality examinations should have in-joke recognition as a central part of the test. If you don't understand the joke you cannot be admitted.

These then are some of the ways in which we construct our own values but there are of course other mechanisms possible. The question which then arises is how are such values transmitted? Later in this book there is a chapter entitled "The Contagious Theory of Behaviour Change" which puts forward an hypothesis to answer this question. It is based on ideas and beliefs being "caught" and transmitted from one person to another through the medium of Transmids. Much more work needs to be done on such non-genetic, contagious mechanisms of behaviour change and attitude formation.

ARE THERE CORE VALUES? So far some possible changes in values have been described and how these might affect clinical practice. The next question is whether such changes are simply cosmetic and not really fundamental in that they do not really change anything and are at the margins of thinking in medical ethics. Has anything fundamentally changed in the last thirty years, the lifetime of my clinical practice? The answer is both yes and no. First then, how has it changed?

The changes. From the examples given above it should be clear that some changes have occurred. So the answer is yes in the sense that there have been real changes both in values and in practice. The best examples would be,

Confidentiality
Genetic screening
Infertility
Cloning and stem cell procedures
Transplantation

They have changed the way in which we think about persons. They have altered some of our concepts and the way we behave.

Core values. It is also clear that some core values have not altered. These are mainly in the area of human rights where, if anything, our affirmation of them has become stronger. Some examples of this would be those taken from the Universal Declaration of Human Rights and might include,

Article 1. All human beings are born free and equal in dignity and rights.
Article 2. Everyone is entitled to all the rights and freedoms set forth in the Declaration, without distinction of any kind such as race, colour, sex, language, religion, political or other opinion, national or social origin, property, birth or other status.
Article 3. Every one has a right to life, liberty and security of person.
Article 5. No one should be subject to torture, or to cruel, inhuman or degrading treatment or punishment.
Article 26. Every one has a right to education.

To this list might be added those most associated with medical ethics, doing no harm (nonmaleficence), a wish to do good (beneficence), the desire to be fair (justice), the wish to help the greater good (utility) and a respect for the individual (autonomy). The "Golden Rule", "Do unto others as they would do to you", "Love thy neighbour" or even the "My mother principle" express in a different way some of these sentiments.

From both of these lists, and there may well be others, it is clear that none of these is specific to doctors. They are all aspects of a democratic society. Are there then any ethical concepts which are specifically medical? Some of these might include the need to be humane, caring and compassionate and to have both calmness and equanimity. (Calman, 1994, Macnaughton, 1996). This raises important issue of doctors and their training. This reflects back on the discussion earlier in this chapter, can such values be taught?

Some consequences. If it is accepted that core values change only very slowly and that there are derived or secondary values which can change more quickly, what are the consequences of this and can a model be developed to assist in our understanding.
Here are some implications.

1. Changes in scope. Some of the changes observed are not real changes, simply changes in the scope of the value. It has broadened or narrowed. The changes in the definition of extra-ordinary means would be an example of this. Or a new technique makes us think more acutely about a particular issue. The introduction of the contraceptive pill which changed attitudes considerably was no more than a technically simpler way of contraception but one which put the onus on women rather than men. Xenotransplantation is in essence no different from the of pig heart valves and indeed the reason for its slow introduction is not an ethical one but a technical one, namely the possibility of viral transmission from the animal to the human. These then are not real changes in values but are a response to new developments in relation to existing ethical issues.

2. The universality of ethical values. There is an assumption that all values need to be agreed by everyone. That abortion is or is not acceptable. That euthanasia is or is not appropriate. This is clearly not the case and in such cases where there is real disagreement it would be difficult to call them "core values". However, they are derived from broader and perhaps more universally agreed values. For example, look again at Article 3 of the Universal Declaration of Human Rights which says "Everyone has a right to life, liberty and security of person." Something that all would agree to. However, in relation to abortion it could be interpreted in two ways. First that the woman has a right to choose an abortion (the liberty argument), or secondly, that the rights of the unborn child also have to be considered pre-eminent (the right to life argument). Hence the secondary or derived nature of some medical ethical points leaving room for individual choice and interpretation. "Thou shalt not kill" is an even clearer statement but is interpreted in many different ways. There are thus legitimate differences in view.

3. Can we then construct a model? This can best be envisaged as a series of concentric rings. The nearer the centre the greater the likelihood that the values will be widely agreed. The further away the derived values become more subject to differences in interpretation. The debate therefore is what constitutes a core value and can they change.

DOES IT MATTER? So what! Does it really matter if values change? Would it make a difference? Would clinical practice really be affected if there were no agreement on values? What are values for anyway? The contention is that it would make a significant difference for a number of reasons, which would include:

1. Patient trust and confidence. At present the trust of our patients is the key to clinical practice. Without this doctors and other health care professionals would have great difficulty in working effectively.

2. Order and disorder. In all societies some form of rules and regulations are required for it to function effectively. Without this chaos can reign. Doctors and others are part of civil society and as such need to be part of its cohesion and substance.

3. Professional standards. This is related to the first point but is closely linked to the concept of a profession (Calman, 1994, Irvine 1997). Professional values bind groups together and provide a way of safeguarding the public. Professional self regulation is thus a consequence of developing core values and also a mechanism for us interpreting changes in the knowledge base, new clinical techniques and changes in the values of society as a whole. Bodies like the General Medical Council and the State Councils, whose role this is, are thus vitally important.

What then are values for? They give coherence to professional groups and give both a sense of purpose and a way of setting and monitoring standards. Without such a code or agreement on ethical values it would not be possible to take into account the rights, wishes and feelings of those in our care and develop the trust required to care compassionately for patients, their families and the community.

SOME CONCLUSIONS

This chapter set out to discuss three broad issues the first of which was how stories might affect our values and beliefs. There is good evidence that they do so and are remarkably powerful forces for change. The second section looked at the teaching and learning of moral issues and showed that literature and story telling did have a role, though clearly not the only way to think through ethical issues. The third section examined the proposition that values in clinical practice could change. Evidence has been presented that they can and that some of these changes relate to the way in which we learn from stories. However, a more in-depth look at such changes suggests that many of these changes have been in secondary or derived values rather than core ones. From the patient's point of view, however, the changes, if any, may be of major importance and need careful thinking through. Professional standards are at the heart of this and must be maintained if patient trust and confidence are to be retained. Values can and do change. We must be vigilant that in making the changes we do not lose what is important in clinical practice, compassion and care.

REFERENCES

Calman,K.C. Downie, R.S, Duthie,M, and Sweeney, B. (1988) Medical Education 22, 488-91.

Calman, K.C. (1994) The profession of medicine. Brit. Med.J. 309, 1140-43.

Calman, K,C. (1997), Literature in the education of the doctor. Lancet, 350, 1622-24

Coles. R. The Call of Stories. Teaching and the moral imagination. 1989 Houghton Miffin Co. Boston.

Downie,R.S. and Macnaughton, R,J. Public Morality and Moral education. In Advances in Bioethics. 1999, 5, 17-29.

Greenhalgh,T and Hurwitz, B. Narrative Based Medicine. Dialogue and discourse in clinical practice. 1998. Brit Med J. Publishing Group, London.

Hawkins, A.N. (1997) Medical Ethics and the Epiphanic Dimension of Narrative. In Nelson, H.L. (Ed) Stories and Their Limits. Narrative approaches to bioethics. Routledge, New York and London.

Huxley, T.H. (1893) Evolution and Ethics. Romanes Lecture. 57pp. (Reissued in Collected Essays, 9 vols.1893-4). London:Macmillan.

Irvine, D. (1997) I. Professionalism and self-regulation in a changing world. Brit. Med J. 314, 1540-2. II. Monitoring good practice, protecting patients from poor performance. Brit. Med,J. 314, 1613-5

Macnaughton, R,J. (1996) Core values: Doctor or everyman? Brit.Med.J. 313, 120-1.

Murray,T.H What do we mean by narrative ethics.1997. Medical Humanities Review, 11, 44-57.

Nelson, H.L. Stories and Their Limits. Narrative approaches to Bioethics. (1997) Routledge, New York and London.

Zeldin, T. An Intimate History of Humanity, 1998, Vintage, London.

APPENDICES

A MEDICAL STUDENT'S LIBRARY

TABLE 1: SIR WILLIAM OSLER

Old and New Testament
Shakespeare
Montaigne
Plutarch's Lives
Marcus Aurelius
Epictetus
Religio Medici Sir Thomas Browne
Don Quixote Cervantes
Emerson
Oliver Wendell Holmes Breakfast Table Series

TABLE 2: BOOKS RECOMMENDED BY DR RICHARD VERNEY (1957)

TITLE	AUTHOR
General	
The Bible	
Anton Chekhov	
Shakespeare's Plays	
Sir Winston Churchill's Writings	
Other Men's Flowers	Field Marshall Lord Wavell
Medical	
A History of Medicine	Douglas Guthrie
The Gold Headed Cane	William Macmichael
John Hunter	Roodhouse Golyne
William Smellie	R W Johnstone
Humphrey Davy	James Kendall
Michael Faraday	James Kendall
The Life of Pasteur	R Vallery-Radot
Lord Lister	Douglas Guthrie
Horae Subsecivae	John Brown
Florence Nightingale	C Woodham Smith

The Life of Sir William Osler   Harvey Cushing
The Writings of Sir William Osler
The Beloved Physician, Sir James Mackenzie   R McNair Wilson
Madame Curie   Eve Curie
Edward Wilson of the Antartic   George Seaver
Berkeley Moynihan, Surgeon   Donald Bateman
The Doctors Mayo   Helen Clapesattle
The Development of Modern Medicine   R H Shryock
My Life and Thought   Albert Schweitzer
The Physician as a Man of Letters, Science & Action   T K Munro
The Quiet Art   Robert Coope

TABLE 3: THE COURSE READING LIST

TITLE	AUTHOR
The Collection of a Library	William Osler
The Citadel	A J Cronin
The Death of Ivan Illich	Lco Tolstoy
Ask the Bloody Horse	
The Poems of Dannie Abse	
Letters from a Stoic	Seneca
The Beloved Physician, Sir James Mackenzie	R McNair Wilson
Rab and his Friends, Horae Subsecivae	John Brown
The Cocktail Party	T S Eliot
Zen and the Art of Motorcycle Maintenance	R Pirsig
On Liberty	J S Mill
Cat on a Hot Tin Roof	Tennessee Williams
The Lumber Room	Saki (H H Munro)
(Collected Stories)	
Death of a Son	Jon Silkin
(Penguin Book of Contemporary Verse)	
Rebecca	Daphne du Maurier
The Doll's House	Henrick Ibsen
Ward 6	Anton Checkhov

TABLE 4: THE 1987 RECOMMENDED LIST - STUDENT SELECTION

TITLE	AUTHOR
Cry, the Beloved Country	Alan Paton
Tess of the d'Urbervilles	Thomas Hardy
The Death of Illich	Leo Tolstoy
Alice in Wonderland	Lewis Carroll
Testament of Youth	Vera Brittain
To Kill a Mocking Bird	Harper Lee
Emma	Jane Austen
Pride and Prejudice	Jane Austen
Silas Marner	George Eliot
Middlemarch	George Eliot
The Lion, the Witch and the Wardrobe	C S Lewis
Nineteen Eighty-Four	George Orwell
The Lord of the Rings	J R R Tolkien
I and Thou	Martin Buber
Jonathan Livingston Seagull	Richard Bach
My God This is Anna	Fynn
Tender is the Night	F Scott Fitzgerald
The Name of the Rose	Umberto Eco
The Colour Purple	Alice Walker
The Little Prince	Antoine de Saint-Exupery
Sunset Song	Lewis Grassic Gibbon
Cal	Bernard MacClaverty
The Aeneid	Virgil

9. The Contagious Theory of Behaviour Change

The Role of The Transmid

"The bacillus of laughter is a difficult bug to isolate: once brought under the microscope it will turn out to be a yeast-like ferment equally useful in making wine or vinegar or bread." *Arthur Koestler in "The Act of Creation."*

There is a sense in which this chapter is the culmination of this book. It brings together the three major themes, storytelling, humour and learning and proposes a mechanism through which they are connected. The proposition has been developed throughout the book using examples, quotations and allusions that change occurs through people, and that ideas, feelings and attitudes are "caught, not taught." It presents the case for a contagious agent, the Transmid, which acts as the vehicle by which ideas are transmitted and that the "story" is the agent itself. The contagious theory of behaviour change is thus based on the analogy of infection and in this chapter this way of thinking will be developed further and some of the possible implications set out.

To begin at the beginning, people change their behaviour for many reasons; and much has been written about the mechanisms involved. One possible mechanism, suggested here, is that people change behaviour because of the way stories affect them and that storytelling is a potentially important way in which this can occur (the effect of the Transmid). We are "changed" by stories, and Gardner (1995) has studied how leaders have used stories as a way of illustrating how behaviour change can be achieved. Perhaps the most well known aspects of this are the parables told by Jesus or the wide range of fables and stories which illustrate particular forms of behaviour and which set a frame of reference for the reader or listener. The early sagas, such as Beowulf (see the discussion in Annexe 1) encourage the listener to adopt particular forms of attitude and those who do not adhere to codes of honour, or who do not believe in dying for a cause, or ferocity in fighting, are condemned. They set the tone for the community and ensure that values are transmitted from generation to generation. This phrase is important as this is precisely the one used to define education in an earlier section of the book, the transmission of values.

One can see these effects of transmission of behaviour in one's children. Many of the traits and features they possess are genetically determined. Others are not. The phrases they use, their mannerisms are "caught" from us, they have been "Transmided". It is salutary to watch yourself in your children as they speak and behave. We "infect" them with our beliefs and values and tell them which football team to support and what catch phrases to use. And yet we can be offended if they reject our pearls of wisdom and behave in a different way. They too will be frustrated when their children reject their own values and beliefs.

This chapter then sets out the hypothesis that in some instances, though not all, people change behaviour because they have been "infected" by the ideas or values of another. It is argued that this "contagion", passed on through "Transmids" (transmitted ideas), can be a very powerful mechanism and may even change the lives of large numbers of people. Story telling is a very powerful force for change. In routine daily life this principle of the contagious theory of change operates on a regular basis. We change our viewing habits, musical tastes, food choices and fashion sense by the stories people tell us. These may be friends, relatives, colleagues or personalities in the media, who tell such good stories about a product or an aspect of lifestyle that we want to change. It is people who bring about change.

The analogy with infection or "contagion" and change is frequently reflected in the literature. For example:

> "It must be borne in mind that surgery, like religion, is caught rather than taught and it follows therefore that the personal relationship between the student and his chief is of greater importance than the details of an educational or training programme." *Sir James Patterson Ross. SGO. 1966-1317-8.*
> "Foul whisperings are abroad. Unnatural deeds
> Do breed unnatural troubles; infected minds
> To their deaf pillows will discharge their secrets;

More needs she the divine than the physician." *Shakespeare in Macbeth*
"The nature of bad news infects the teller." *Shakespeare in Anthony and Cleopatra*

People are thus the agents of transmission of change and in common use the phrase "Caught not taught" as a way of thinking about teaching illustrates the point clearly.

The concept, therefore, is not new and has been raised on many occasions. In Richard Dawkin's book, "The Selfish Gene" (1976) he concludes by suggesting another form of transmission of traits, this time by imitation. He calls this memes, shortened from the word "mimeme", to imitate. Others have picked this concept up and there has been a spate of books on memes and related topics. These include "The Virus of the Mind. The New Science of the Meme." by Richard Brodie (1996), "Thought Contagion. How Beliefs Spread Through Society," by Aaron Lynch (1996), "Consciousness Explained" (1991) and "Darwin's Dangerous Idea" by Daniel Dennett (1995). The most recent of these is "The Meme Machine" by Susan Blackmore. Each of these picks up the concept that ideas can be transmitted and in essence jump from brain to brain. The mechanism by which this is achieved is unknown but it is regularly pointed out that DNA was not discovered as the mechanism of genetic transmission until decades after Darwin. We must await, therefore, a molecular explanation of the way in which non-genetic transmission of behaviour occurs. The link between such memes and learning is of course also made, as indeed it is with humour.

Susan Blakemore at the start of her book says "The theme of this book (The Meme Machine) is that what makes us different is our ability to imitate". This present book has the same function though it assumes that in many instances stories are the mechanism. However, it goes beyond the meme hypothesis in that not all changes in behaviour are as a result of imitation. Learning is more than that and the transmission of ideas is much more than simply doing things the way that others do. It is for this reason that in this book the word "Transmid" is used to describe the mechanism by which ideas, behaviour, knowledge and information are transmitted from one person to another. This can be done personally or through the medium of books or other types of media. Transmids are therefore words (or word substitutes) used singly or in combination, in a way which affects others, or effects change. The possible biological characteristics of the Transmid will be discussed later in this chapter.

Learning is the most obvious way by which the Transmid operates. The information about how to drive a car, how to carry out an appendectomy, or how to break bad news are all part of this. It is part of teaching. We learn how to do, and to teach, by watching others, reading and trying things out for ourselves. Some of this is undoubtably imitation but once again it is more than this. In a similar way the use of humour in teaching and learning, or in our daily lives, represents other ways in which ideas and behaviour are transmitted.

How then can this analogy be developed further? How can we better define the characteristics of the agent of change, the Transmid and the process Transmidering? Examples from the field of infectious disease will be used to illustrate the concept.

1. Virulence. Some people seem better than others at conveying and delivering a message. High virulence people are able to tell a clear story with high impact. You want to hear and you want to believe. Others, low virulence people, have less credibility and power. They are not so good at telling the tale in a convincing and effective way. Some organisms are symbiotic or commensals and are thus present without any obvious effect, though essential in their own way. Their impact is small and this might be seen as equivalent to the routine and humdrum aspects of life. We hear but we don't listen to the background noise unless something special is told to us by someone special. The Transmid then becomes operative. Virulent organisms need to be transmitted by vectors who are the people who transmit the story. Even a powerful story may not be effective if it is delivered inappropriately.

2. Superbugs. Such individuals often have immense power to change people. They are frequently high profile individuals in positions of responsibility. They may have come from an obscure background but because of the force of their convictions and the power of their personality they change the fate and behaviour of millions. Once they have infected a person or a group of people the message is spread onwards by disciples or acolytes who maintain the integrity of the message. This phenomenon, sometimes known as social amplification, can affect a very large group of people very quickly indeed. Look how rapidly fashions change in children's toys just before Christmas.

3. Resistance. The hypothesis assumes that, as for infection, the "soil" must be fertile in order that the individual can be changed, for the contagion to spread. This is not necessarily true. Resistance or even immunity may occur. The message may not be received, the individual may be entirely immune to the agent, or the timing of the contagion may not be right. The soil might not be fertile and no change may occur. Breaking down the resistance may be difficult, but might occur at particular points of time when the person is especially vulnerable. Sudden changes of behaviour (alcohol cessation may occur in this way), or a life event of some magnitude (a sudden serious illness) may be sufficient to damage the immunity and allow change to occur. For example, in spite of fact that the vast majority of the population know that smoking is harmful to health, 25% continue to smoke. It is not because they have not heard, or indeed not even understood, it must be because the product is addictive, and that the value of continuing to smoke is greater to the individual, than stopping. The timing of the Transmid infection is thus critical.

The size of the infective dose may also be critical. Small amounts of the same message over a period of time may breed familiarity and contempt and the message may be lost. Tolerance or immunity may even be developed. Under these circumstances it is extremely difficult to reverse the process, unless the immunity is broken down.

4. Routes of Transmission. If this hypothesis is to be plausible and the metaphor valid there must be routes of transmission. In this instance words and feelings (written, spoken or delivered in many other ways) gain access via the senses, especially sight, hearing and touch; they are transmided. Each of these senses is a route of entry. Emotions and feelings are also important. The contagious agent must interact with one of them or be sufficiently virulent to engender change.

The stories used (the Transmids) may be verbal and non verbal. Actions, attitudes and observed behaviour may be just as powerful as reading a book or listening to a story. In clinical terms the hidden curriculum in medical education would be a good example of this. The attitude and behaviour of senior doctors on ward rounds, in clinics, in operating theatres, is rapidly transmitted to students or junior staff. Communication

skills can be directly observed and subsequently copied, for good or ill.
The skills of doctors are also transmitted in this way as juniors watch their
seniors in theatre, in the clinic, or at the bedside.

5 Good and Bad Organisms. So far it has been assumed that the contagious
theory only works for good. That change is always to be welcomed and
leads to a better life or way of behaviour. Clearly this is not necessarily true.
Bad behaviour can also be transmided in the same way. Smoking, alcohol,
drugs, dietary habits can be changed in an adverse way as well as for the
good. There is no discrimination with the contagious agent, the Transmid,
it must be active or it will die out. Bad and good habits need to be sustained.

In this way it differs in concept from education but not in mechanism.
Education always has associated with it a value for good. It is a beneficial
process. In the contagious theory of behaviour change the alteration can
go either way in the same way as training also can. One can be trained to
do things badly.

6. Acute Changes in Behaviour. In many instances behaviour changes
slowly. Our tastes and hobbies change with age, for example, over a period
of years. With the contagious theory, however, change can occur very
rapidly indeed, over a few hours, suggesting a remarkably acute process.
The effects of the Transmid can be seen very quickly. The best examples
of this are with religious conversion, a process which can occur within
moments. Other examples would be in the giving up of alcohol or drugs,
often at a very vulnerable part in one's life. The mechanism for this
suggests a sudden, fulminating change with an agent (the Transmid) which
is able to change a complete personality.

7. Latency or dormancy. Sometimes an infectious agent settles in a tissue or
organ and remains latent or dormant for some time, often for many years.
Herpes infections would be very good examples of this. Something
triggers them off and they become virulent and active once again. So it is
with ideas sown many years ago which may surface and come alive.
Forgotten in the depths of the memory they come into the consciousness
and then may affect the behaviour, feelings or attitudes of the individual.
The concept of "epiphany" fits well into this section. The idea may have

been there for some time but suddenly, "the penny drops", the idea or the solution, is "seen" and the "Eureka" response occurs. There is a sudden outbreak caused by an event or another Transmid.

THE IMPLICATIONS If this hypothesis has any credibility what are its implications and how could it be tested? The hypothesis suggests that people change because of the impact of stories (verbal and non verbal) told by one person and affecting another. The implications are not new.

(a) The character of the person telling the story is critical. They need credibility, an opportunity to tell the story, and they need to be good at it. If the story cannot be told, or there is no audience, there can be no change. Exposure to one of the senses is essential for the Transmid to operate. The range of ways in which stories can be told and the multiple media available mean that very large audiences could be affected rapidly. This is reflected in clinical practice in that the range of information and the access to stories is now enormous.

(b) The nature of the story is fundamental and is perhaps the most important feature. The message, the language, the power, the impact of the story are critical and probably more important than the teller of the tale. Its credibility, realism, imagery, linkage to familiar concepts, places and people are probably most relevant.

In medical terms the story needs to have a background and a setting to which the listener can relate. It needs to use words and concepts which can be readily understood. It should be grounded in reality - real patients, real problems. Understanding of the issues is critical and the level of knowledge important. The development of problem based learning and the increasing use of real patients and of carefully developed case histories is part of this process.

(c) The presentation of the story. In some instances good stories can emerge rapidly and effortlessly. For many people, however, putting together a story, getting its sequence correct, improving its relevance, making it live, can take time and a great deal of work. Searching for analogies, illustrations, quotations, anecdotes to make the story memorable can be difficult and time consuming. To find, at last, the one slide or story which will capture a whole idea or concept can be an exciting moment on the part of the storyteller. It is part of the creative process. The story may need to be modified, extended and reviewed with time as the clarity of the message increases. That is part of the skill and the spell of the storyteller.

The process of research is often similar. It begins with an idea, a journal article, an observation, or a story told by someone, perhaps a patient or a colleague. The idea begins to infect thinking and following discussions with others, and a check of the literature, this may then suggest a new and original way of writing a new story which then has to be tested. If the research comes to fruition and the idea is found to be a good one then others will be told of the story. For those who write research grants on a regular basis it is the first part of this, convincing the Research Body that the story is plausible, which is most difficult!

Sometimes the form of a story emerges with time and with conversations with others whose stories blend and integrate with the original one. In visual terms it is akin to Michaelangelo's block of stone with no form or shape. However, with work, skill and imagination a figure emerges from the block, clear and identifiable. Basil Bunting in the "First Book of Odes", uses a similar analogy with words. He calls the process, "the sharp tool paring away waste and the forms cut out of mystery". It is a most powerful process and requires very hard work and skill. Eventually the Transmid is ready to operate, to transmid knowledge and information.

(d) The nature of the listener. Listeners can be of several types. First, there are the wise listeners (sometimes called professors or opinion leaders) whose task is to interpret the story. If there is to be a change in behaviour or attitude such individuals are key to the diffusion of the idea or knowledge and of any change in practice. If they can be convinced, others will follow (they are sometimes called the early adopters) and they become the disciples.

The second group are the majority who on listening to the tale may wish to change but at the same time will need a lead. They are busy and need to be convinced but will change if the new idea is of value. The final group are those who are very difficult to infect (the laggards). Here the Transmid falls on stony ground and such individuals can provide, for many years, foci of resistance.

Such groups have, of course, been well described elsewhere in the literature (Rogers, 1995) associated with the concept of diffusion of innovation. The Transmid hypothesis fits it well. Thus, in a very significant aspect of medical practice, the implementation of evidence-based change in clinical work, both the role of the story as well as a review of the literature may have a place. From the point of view of the contagious hypothesis the important features would be leadership and an effective story told by credible people.

(e) The nature of the environment. Even virulent organisms can be overcome by other infectious agents, as the analogy of the bacteriophage shows, or by antibacterial agents. An individual may be infected by a Transmid (by a colleague, at a course, by a visit to another clinical practice) but on return to base may be prevented, by a series of barriers, in practising the new behaviour or technique. The attitudes and behaviours of others can be powerful antimicrobial agents and prevent infection and dissemination. The process of sterilisation is real. The social context of change needs to be considered at all stages as the infectious analogy demonstrates.

In essence these attributes relate to what good teachers do and such individuals occur in all walks of life. While it may be true that some are more gifted than others it is possible for all to improve their teaching skills. This is perhaps one of the most important implications, that all those who teach can do it even better by careful preparation and presentation of the story. Such teaching events do not just happen, they take time, effort, rehearsal and are improved by experience and feedback from the learners (listeners). Good storytellers continually modulate their story to reflect the audience and its interests. Good storytellers respond to the audience and draw from the audience sources of examples and lessons. They use the Transmids already in the audience to increase the power of the learning environment .

Teaching, like story telling is a highly professional activity

SOME FURTHER THOUGHTS. From these discussions two further implications arise. First what is the mechanism of action of the Transmid? And second, how can we improve the potency of its action?

1. The mechanism of action of the Transmid. There has been no discussion so far on the mechanism of the infection. How does it happen, how is it remembered? What is the equivalent of the DNA in genetic transmission? How do they jump from brain to brain? How is it copied? What is it which gives the instructions for carrying out a change in behaviour and which affect this in such a way as to sustain the change for some time? It needs to be replicated and to be able to do this faithfully and effectively. The terms meme or Transmid have been used to describe this potential agent, the effective agent which transmits behaviour, ideas and values. It is transmitted by words and deeds and some people are more able to disseminate Transmids than others.

The molecular mechanism is at this stage quite unclear. However, the developments in neurobiology and of our understanding of brain function which have occurred in the last decade will help in the process. We need to define the characteristics of the Transmid which allow it to reach the brain, be replicated, sustained and be copied faithfully. It then needs to be able to be passed on to others or its value is lost. There is a major research project in that statement. There are, however, a number of experimental models which could be used to test some of the mechanisms, the most obvious of which is in the process of learning. This could be the learning of almost anything, but the undergraduate experience which involves knowledge, attitudes and skills would seem to be an ideal one to explore.

A second model would be that of "conversion" which describes any experience (not necessarily a religious one) in which behaviour changes rapidly. There must be many more lessons still to be learned from that process. And finally there is humour and how it makes people laugh and, on occasions, feel better. The laughter clinic is not just an idea to be scorned, there may be some real value in it. We could learn a great deal from the observation of people who have been stimulated in a particular kind of way.

Another question is where do new ideas "Transmids" come from? How do new ideas arise? Reference has already been made to the effort which is required to generate new ideas. It is an exhausting though exhilarating task. Brain work is required which needs a source of energy or food. It is interesting that in the work of Freud and others on humour the concept of work is constantly referred to. Ideas may come from others or from within ourselves if we have the curiosity to find out more. The brain needs to be kept in trim, it needs a regular fitness programme. It needs to be constantly exercised by Transmids, to stimulate and excite. Like any other kind of training programme this needs time and effort.

2. Improving the effectiveness of Transmids. Although we cannot yet describe the mechanism of action of the agent, this should not stop us from looking at ways of improving learning and teaching. As has been described in an earlier chapter there are many ways in which the knowledge we have could be used now to make things better. That is the task of those who have the responsibility to ensure quality in education. From a medical perspective the situation is even clearer. We know that more patients could be treated more effectively, by more doctors, more of the time. Some will of course say that this is a financial issue and some of it is. But much of it is not about money but about attitudes and a willingness to change. The role of the Transmid and the leader, the person who can transmit knowledge and ideas to others, has never been more important.

CONCLUSIONS

This chapter is at the heart of the book. It discusses a mechanism by which learning, humour and stories come together and suggests that those who can tell good stories, and thus send out Transmids, are very important for the profession as a whole. We need leadership and a culture which is willing to accept and be challenged by change. Not for its own sake, but for the benefit of patients and the public.

REFERENCES

Blackmore, S. The Meme Machine. 1999. Oxford University Press.

Brodie, R. The Virus of the Mind: The new science of the meme 1996. Seatle. WA. Integral Press.

Dawkins, R. The Selfish Gene. 1976. Oxford University Press. (Revised Edition with additional material, 1989)

Dennett, D. Consciousness Explained. 1991. Little Brown, Boston. MA.

 Dennett,D. Darwin's Dangerous Idea.1995. Penguin, London.

Lynch, A. Thought Contagion. How belief spreads through society. 1996. Basic Books, New York

Gardner, H. Leading Minds. An anatomy of leadership. 1995. Harper Collins, London.

Rogers, E.M. The Diffusion of Innovation. 1995. 4th Edition. Free Press of Glencoe. New York

10. Endpiece

"Till on the drowsy page the light grows dim
And doubtful slumber half supplies the theme
While antique shapes of knight and giant grim
Damsel and dwarf, in long procession gleam
And the romancer's tale becomes the reader's dream."

Sir Walter Scott in "Harold the Dauntless."

The introduction of Scott's great narrative poem, "Harold the Dauntless" describes the essence of this book wonderfully well: the "romancer's tale becomes the reader's dream", the connection between the author and the reader, the tale and the listener. As the whole of the introduction to "Harold the Dauntless" is in praise of books and reading it is reproduced at length as Annexe 2. For readers in the North of England a perhaps more familiar section of this poem is the one which describes Durham Cathedral as:

"Grey towers of Durham....
Well yet I love thy mix'd and massive piles
Half church of God, half castle 'gainst the Scot."

The key line of the poem (romancer's tale to reader's dream) uses the same imagery as Osler's phrase, "mind to mind" in relation to textbooks, as it is a process which unites two minds (the writer and the reader) which are separated only by print. The reading sets off ideas, dreams and fires the imagination. As has been covered throughout the book, and especially chapter 9, it is suggested that this process is mediated via Transmids.

In this Endpiece the three themes of the book (storytelling, humour and learning) are brought together once again with some further reflections. The objective of the book was to try to find a link between the three and the Transmid hypothesis is the culmination of this. There are, however, a number of other consequences which flow from this general conclusion.

Clinical practice. The obvious lessons are for greater skills in listening and interpreting the stories that patients tell us. Of taking a broader holistic view of the (his)tory and of seeing patients and their families as part of a wider ecological system. Identifying their place in the nature of things and in seeing them in a public health perspective.

Part of this is the building up of trust between the patient and the doctor. This is a process which can take time yet may be the most valuable part of the relationship. Without trust the ability to discuss difficult problems openly, and as equals, is unlikely to be possible. Making sense of uncertainty is one of the most difficult aspects of the doctor's role but it is made easier if trust exists.

This close relationship is well described in Martin Buber's book, "I and Thou" (Clark, Edinburgh, 1958) in which human relationships are said to be of two types. The first, the "I and you" relationship, would be the normal kind between two people who do not know each other well, courteous and formal, and associated with respect for feelings and circumstances. It is the master-pupil relationship, or that between the customer and the client. It is the second type of relationship which is more interesting. Buber's "I and Thou" category is deeper and much more fulfilling. He also describes it as a sharing of hearts. It is a relationship akin to love in which the two individuals can do without speech, in that everything can be unspoken, but understood. In dealing with very ill patients in whom there is a real involvement in their well-being this can occur and is one of the privileges of being a doctor. In the long term family links in general practice a similar type of relationship can occur. Henry James' book "The Wings of the Dove" describes such a relationship between patient and doctor.

It might be going too far to link these thoughts with healing skills, healing in this sense being related to wholeness and not to curing. The doctor, and many other health professionals, do have a role in this healing process, in helping others to be whole again. The story and the Transmid can have a part in this.

Reference has been made on several occasions to quality of life, a concept which is difficult to define. Some time ago (Calman, K.C. Quality of life in cancer patients. An hypothesis. J. Med. Ethics. 1984, 10, 124-7.) it was proposed that quality of life measured the difference between hopes and aspirations and reality. It was the gap between the two which reflected quality and the quality of life improves if we can narrow the gap. It is interesting to re-visit this in relation to storytelling, learning and humour. In each instance if there is a positive response then quality of life is likely to improve. For example learning something new and useful, hearing a good story, and having some fun and laughter. The gap narrows. On the other hand the reverse may well be the case. We are unable to learn and keep up to date. We hear only distressing stories and there is no laughter in our lives. The gap widens. Some of this we can influence ourselves, other aspects are out of our control. The gap matters to us all and the need to tell and listen to stories is very much part of this.

One of the important sections of the book was to make the link between anecdote and evidence. There is no contradiction between the two, they are both necessary and required if the full picture is to be revealed. The medical student of the future will not only require an in-depth knowledge of molecular biology and genetics but skills in the human aspects of medicine. This book, emphasising the relevance of stories, is thus not an attack on the evidence-based approach, rather the contrary, recognising as it does connection between the two.

Ethical issues are of increasing interest in clinical practice and rightly so. Stories can add to our understanding of the moral problems which might arise. They allow us to see such problems in a different way and to personalise the issues from the stories which patients tell us.

Medical stories, serious and humourous, are fascinating and add so much to our enjoyment of being a doctor. We learn through stories and they have much to teach us. The stories about medical students show what a wonderful experience it was and hopefully still is. Add to this the wide range of stories in the literature of the world and the stories patients tell and there is a lifelong quest for fun and enjoyment.

Stories and conversation. The salons of the 18th century had, as their primary purpose, the facilitation of conversation. They were places where a range of people could be invited, not for their wealth or position, but because they had something to say. This rather rosy picture of the scene has a direct parallel in medical practice today. There is a need for doctors, and others, to be able to talk to each other. As the pace of change grows, so it becomes even more important. Exchanging e-mail is not the only way of communicating and it remains important that there are times and places where conversation between two or more people and an exchange of stories can occur. The Medical Society, now under threat in many places, performed this function, bringing specialists and generalists together. Loneliness can occur in doctors as well as others and the need to talk and share triumphs and failures is important. The wonderful phrase in "Beowulf", the "word-hoard", is relevant. We all have things to say, word-hoards to discharge and empty, and we need someone to listen. Such conversations can act as catalysts for change and improvement. The definition of a catalyst being a substance which effects change and is not destroyed in the process.

Stories give us roots and through these roots stability, nourishment and a capacity for growth. They anchor us in the past and the present and help us to develop towards the future. We need opportunities to tell our stories and to listen to those of others, to be affected and infected with their thoughts and ideas; the role of the Transmid.

Leadership, stories and role models. One of the most potent aspects of storytelling is in the establishment of leadership. Good leaders tell good stories and their power, at least in part, rests on this ability. It must be supplemented, of course, by knowledge and other skills but the ability to describe where you want to go, and how to get there, is critical. This is where power resides, in the capacity to convince others that your story is likely to be more effective than that of someone else. A study of the history of medicine is instructive in this respect. Many of the "greats" in medicine, the leaders of the past and of the present, those who took the profession to new heights, or who discovered new ways of diagnosis or treatment, had great stories to tell. In one sense the history of medicine is also a synthesis of the book. It brings storytelling and learning together and shows how changes in behaviour and action can occur.

Research. The research agenda which flows from this book is a very full one. In education, learning and humour, there are many questions which remain unanswered. For example, the interest in humour is not just in making people laugh, others can do that. It is in the consequences of laughter and the resultant happiness which is of interest. If humour does really make us feel better and there is considerable evidence that it does, how can we exploit this to improve quality of life and well-being? What is the mechanism and how can it be better understood? Is there really a "sense of humour" equivalent to our other senses and if so why not try to understand it and benefit from such an understanding?

As our insights into the workings of the brain grow and the techniques for investigation expand, so the possibilities for research increase. The experimental models are not difficult to find and in a University setting the undergraduate population geared to learning is an ideal group. At least two different situations could be envisaged for study. The first relates to the acquisition of a new subject, of which language is the most obvious. Here is an experimental setting in which an entirely new knowledge base is to be learned, often with no previous background. Much is already being done in this area, but often in individual disciplines, and this is a topic which would benefit from a multi-disciplinary approach. The second relates to theatre and the production and direction of plays. In this experimental setting not only is there learning of the lines but of the learning of much higher order issues such as feelings and emotions. Why could this not be used to investigate the learning process as it occurs within the brain? Other examples might include the learning of a musical instrument or of a new clinical skill.

An interesting aspect of this topic is the "work" which is required to achieve learning, and even more so in terms of creativity. Freud's "dream-work" would be the analogy. We feel tired and exhausted after such an effort though physically we may have done nothing but sit, think, and write. We talk about the energy required to carry out the process and relate this to other types of energy. In engineering terms entropy is the tendency to sink into chaos. Energy is needed to constantly keep the system organised and functioning. Perhaps there is something which might be called "neural entropy", which constantly requires energy to keep our ideas coming and to organise our learning. The energy may keep our concept maps intact.

In Scotland in the 18th century there grew up an interest in what was called the "Commonsense" school of philosophy. It concentrated on how all the senses worked together to achieve a synthesis which then resulted in "commonsense". The term has been rather overused recently and its original meaning has changed somewhat. However it remains a powerful concept, as it balances the senses and provides a judgement and an overview of the appropriate course of action. If to the five senses a sense of humour is also added then the idea becomes complete. It is about quality of life, of balance in living and ultimately happiness, however that is defined by the individual.

Two other concepts were raised in the book which might benefit from repeating here. The first is the concept of curiosity, an essential attribute of the doctor. It allows the doctor or the student to become an explorer and adventurer. To go where no one has gone before and to seek out new frontiers. If this sounds rather like Star Trek it is meant to. There is still a human need to do something different and many of the opportunities to explore continents and countries are now limited. But there remains a whole domain of intellectual discovery to be explored. This must be part of the work of the doctor of the future.

The second topic is that of epiphany, the process by which something is revealed as a sudden event. We "see" things and understand things sometimes with a flash of insight. How is this done, and what is the mechanism? The Eureka response is similar in learning, creativity and in understanding a joke. It suddenly "dawns" on us (what a splendid analogy) that a new fact or concept fits in and changes our thinking. It is a remarkable process and it would be good if we could make sense of its mechanism and use it more frequently.

A concluding paragraph. The objective of this book, to use an alternative frame of reference, was to explore happiness and to see how learning, storytelling and humour could contribute to it. These are all subjects which are fundamental to our quality of life and how we cope with ourselves and the world around us. It is important that doctors remain explorers and adventurers, seeking out new ways of improving health, quality of care and of managing illness. It is hoped that the discussions have gone some way towards improving our understanding of happiness and to have spread a little of it about in to process.

Annexe 1
A Holiday Reading Interlude
A Review of Some Old Tales

"The leader of the troop unlocked his word hoard;"
Seamus Heaney. "Beowolf"

In the summer of 1999, during the writing of this volume, five specific books or poems were chosen for re-reading. They were not chosen at random, as all had "tale" or "sagas" in their title. They were read at the mid-point of writing and thinking about this book and tested the thoughts and concepts developed to that stage. It is recognised that not everyone will be interested in what others read on holiday but it was a fascinating exercise. Some new books were also read but that is another story.

One further word of introduction, this part of the book was not designed as an academic exercise in criticism or analysis but for enjoyment and relaxation. The comments and the quotations are therefore not to be seen as the definitive guide to a particular collection of stories and tales. They are personal and reflective comments from the beach and the aeroplane. On previous occasions the author has used similar holiday events to request reading material from staff, successfully doing this for several years in the Department of Health when a series of splendid books were suggested by medical staff following a round-robin e-mail. Perhaps an idea to be taken up elsewhere by others.

The Collections chosen were Aesop's Fables, Penguin Edition 1998; Grimms' Fairy Tales, Penguin Popular Classics Edition, 1996; The Anglo-Saxon World, World's Classics Edition, which contains "Beowulf", Oxford University Press, 1994; The Canterbury Tales by Geoffrey Chaucer, Penguin Edition, 1977; and Tam O'Shanter; A Tale by Robert Burns, using the Oxford Book of Narrative Verse, 1983. All had been read before but not in the current wider context of story telling. In late 1999 the Seamus Heaney translation of Beowulf was published and it has been used here to contrast some of the language in the

World's Classics Edition. These tales were chosen not only because they were
well known but because they had endured many centuries of re-telling and thus
might have qualities and features which were distinctive. They are survivors.

1. Aesop's Fables. These fables were written and collected by Aesop in early
   6th century Greece. The Penguin Edition of them (Penguin Books, 1998,
   Edited by O and R Temple) makes it clear that some were from other parts
   of the ancient world, such as Libya or Egypt and that they served as a
   series of oral stories before being written down. They were often quoted
   at dinner parties and were referred to by Aristophanes, Plato and Aristotle.
   As the editor suggests they were used as a kind of "joke book" and could
   be used to select a story to fit an occasion. Reading through them many
   seem appropriate to be used in contemporary teaching and speech
   making. Here are three, the morals are those from the text, with one
   obvious exception.

The North Wind and the Sun. The North Wind and the Sun had a
contest of strength. They decided to allot the palm of victory to whichever
of them could strip the clothes off a traveller.

The North Wind tried first. He blew violently. As the man clung on to his
clothes, the North Wind attacked him with greater force. But the man,
uncomfortable from the cold, put on more clothes. So disheartened, the
North Wind left him to the Sun.

The Sun now shone moderately and the man removed his extra cloak.
Then the sun darted beams which were more scorching until the man, not
being able to withstand the heat, took off his clothes and went for a dip in a
nearby river.

Moral: This fable shows that persuasion is often more effective than
violence.

Zeus and the Men. Having made men, Zeus entrusted Hermes with
pouring over them some intelligence. Hermes making equal quantities
poured each man his portion. Thus it happened that short men, covered

by their portion, became sensible people, but the tall men, not being covered by all the mixture, had less sense than the others.

Moral: Would you believe that I'm small!

The Lioness and the Vixen. A vixen criticised a lioness for only ever bearing one child. "Only one" she said, "but a lion".

Moral: Do not judge merit by quantity, but by worth.

These are just three of a wide range of stories which can be used to illustrate various aspects of life. Other well known ones include the "Tortoise and the Hare", the "Town Mouse and the Country Mouse" and the 'Man who Promised the Impossible". I suspect most doctors have a similar collection of stories, some humourous and some clinical, with which to expand and illuminate talks or clinical meetings. Aesop's "one liners" were well used in their day. Watching colleagues at dinners noting down good stories suggests that the practice is still alive and well.

2. Grimms' Fairy Tales. These tales were collected in the 18th century by two very dedicated brothers who spent their lives listening to, and recording, the stories, tales and legends. Their work has endured several centuries and includes such standards as Little Red Riding Hood, Rumplestiltskin and Tom Thumb. The stories are full of magic, kings, queens, princes and princesses alongside shepherds and old men and women. There are talking animals and birds, strange creatures and mysterious woods, castles and cottages. The stories are about human emotions and feelings such as pride, greed, love, ambition, hate and fear. Good always triumphs and badness is generally punished. The stories are full of moral teaching. They help consider what is right and what is wrong. There are no greys, only black and white.

   Such fairy stories have deep and lasting psychological significance and they have been well recorded and analysed by Bruno Bettleheim in his book "The Uses of Enchantment" (1976). They deal with emotions and feelings and, more so than Aesop, set out right and wrong, in perhaps too clear a way for us nowadays. They are, however, more than just children's stories but represent hidden values which extend across generations and cultures.

From a medical point of view they have little direct parallel. However, the importance of values and moral attitudes in medicine is as strong as ever. We are unlikely to use these stories in the teaching of medical ethics, they give only one view of a problem or a human feeling. They do, however, make it plain that clarification of one's own views are important if we are to understand the feelings of others.

3. Boewulf and the Anglo-Saxon Literature. These great sagas provide a different view of the world. They are realistic yet at the same time deal with mythical beings such as dragons and strange beasts. They tell stories of great heroism and courage. They show what was expected of a man, to put his honour above all and to respond to the call of friendship. To deny this would be to commit a serious breach of kinship and would bring disgrace. They describe a code of behaviour, the ideal towards which every man should aim. The legends of the ones who have gone before are honoured and their stories retold to influence future generations.

Beowulf is a stirring story of great courage and sacrifice. Having killed the monster as a young man and achieved great fame another task awaits him in his later years which leads to his death, though he also manages to destroy the dragon. It is a powerful story. You can feel the tension and the pain and it is a story which is both horrific and memorable. Some quotations from the Oxford Classics Edition (1984) illustrate some of these points more vividly.

> "I have also heard men say this monster
> Is so reckless he spurns the use of weapons.
> Therefore (so that Hygelac, my Lord
> May rest content over my conduct) I deny myself
> The use of a sword and broad yellow shield
> In battle; but I shall fight for our lives."

and

> "Beowulf, the son of Ecgtheow answered
> do not grieve, wise Hrothgar Better each man
> should avenge his friend than deeply mourn."

and

> "Beowulf trusted in his own strength,
> the might of his hand. So must any man
> who hopes to gain long lasting fame
> in battle; he must risk life regardless."

and again

> "This is not your undertaking, nor is it
> possible for any man but me alone
> to pit his strength against the gruesome one,
> and perform great deeds. I will gain the gold
> by daring, or else battle, dread destroyer
> of life, will lay claim to your Lord."

The translation by Seamus Heaney, which won the Booker Prize for 1999, is a fluid and vivid achievement. In the Introduction he emphasises his Irish and Celtic inheritance and illustrates how some of the language has been chosen. Two quotations, which are particularly striking, are related here and compared to the World Classics Edition.

The first comes from the first few lines

> "The man who wins renown
> Will always prosper among any people."

And from the Heaney translation

> "Behaviour that is admired
> Is the path to power among people everywhere."

What a statement about leadership and the need to tell good stories! The second extract comes from early on in the poem.

> "The man of highest standing, the leader of that troop,
> Unlocked his hoard of words, answered him."

And from the Heaney translation

> "The leader of the troop unlocked his word-hoard;
> The distinguished one delivered his answer."

Unlocking the "word-hoard" is a splendid turn of phrase, and one which could almost be the title of this book and is of course quoted at the beginning of this chapter. It is what we do when we converse, tell stories or jokes and teach. Each of us has a "word-hoard" and we should open it regularly and use it. Like the chemical catalyst or the enzyme, it will transform other things and not be used up in the process.

These extracts illustrate the culture of the Anglo-Saxon. Courage, daring and a life for others. Beowulf and similar sagas give guidance on how to behave, how to deal with problems, how to choose what is right. Such tales glorify the hero and encourage the story to be told so that others may benefit.

From a medical point of view stories do the same. They set standards in clinical behaviour, set out what is acceptable, and what is not and provide the hidden agenda in medical practice. They establish what is important and who is important. They set the road for others to follow. They establish the culture and the rehearsing of the histories of the great ones can be uplifting and visionary. They can be just as powerful as Beowulf was to the early Anglo-Saxons in determining our ideas and behaviour. Leadership is just as important in medicine as it was in Beowulf's era.

4. The Canterbury Tales. These tales are altogether different from the other three collections. They deal with real people in real time and describe in remarkable detail the lives of a motley group of people who are on their way to Canterbury on a pilgrimage. In Chaucer's own words,

> "Some nine and twenty in a company
> Of sundry fold happening then to fall
> In fellowship, and they were pilgrims all
> That towards Canterbury meant to ride."

They leave from the Tabard Inn in Southwark and their host persuades them all
to tell each other a story on the way. The stories themselves are funny, crude,
serious and illuminating. But perhaps the most interesting part is where Chaucer
introduces the characters in the Prologue. They are masterly succinct case
histories, as good as any on a ward round. Here are few selections.

The Nun

> "At meat her manners were well taught withal;
> No morsel from her lips did she let fall,
> Nor dipped her fingers in the sauce too deep;
> But she could carry a morsel up and keep
> The smallest drop from falling on her breast.
> For courtliness she had a special zest
> And she would wipe her upper lip so clean
> That not a trace of grease was to be seen."

The Oxford Cleric

> "His only care was study, and indeed
> He never spoke a word more than was need
> Formal at that, respectful in the extreme
> Short to the point, and lofty in his theme.
> A tone of moral virtue filled his speech
> And gladly would he learn and gladly teach."

The Doctor

> "Yet he was rather close as to expenses
> And kept the gold he won in pestilences
> Gold stimulates the heart, or so we're told
> He therefore had a special love of gold."

The Summoner

> "There was a Summoner with us at that Inn
> His face on fire, like a cherubim,

For he had carbuncles. His eyes were narrow.
He was as hot and lecherous as a sparrow.
Black scabby brows he had, and a thin beard
Children were afraid when he appeared.
No quicksilver, lead ointment, tartar creams,
No brimstone, no boracic, so it seems,
Could make a salve that he had the power to bite
Clean up or cure his whelks of knobby white."

What marvellous clinical descriptions, and in verse too. The power of such pen portraits is very real. So indeed are real life clinical descriptions at the bedside and ward round which it is our privilege to be part of each day. Memorable and real they give a further link to medical story telling and the importance of the anecdote and narrative. It is not a difficult skill to acquire and to use for both teaching and to stimulate curiosity, the beginnings of clinical research. As usual there is one proviso, that the anecdote about a specific patient should always be checked against the literature as a whole and the particular clinical problem placed in context. Chaucer's nun may not have been typical of all nuns, or the doctor of all doctors, but they provide a fascinating starting point for research into medieval medicine and the church.

The final phrase used here in the quotations by the Cleric could also be our watchword, "And gladly would he learn and gladly teach". Teaching is a privilege and something which as doctors we should see as one of our responsibilities. It has been since Hippocratic times and should always continue to be so.
Tam O'Shanter. This a tale which had been read many times and enjoyed. It is very quotable and one needs only to think of

"Nae man can tether time or tide
The hour approaches Tam maun ride."
Or,
"But pleasures are like poppies spread:
You seize the flower its bloom is shed;
Or like the snowfall in the river,
A moment white then gone forever."

It begins in festive mood at the end of a market day. Tam goes to the pub to meet his old friend Souter Johnny, "his ancient trusty drouthy crony". The first few lines set the tone.

> "As market days are wearing late
> And folk begin to tak the gate
> While we sit bousing at the nappy
> Getting fou and unco happy."

Tam begins to enjoy the evening and he and the landlady flirt a little and the old stories are re-told.

> "The landlady and Tam grew gracious
> Wi' secret favours, sweet and precious
> The Souter tauld his queerest stories
> The landlord's laugh was ready chorus."

Outside a storm is brewing and Tam has to ride home through the dark Ayrshire countryside to face his wife. So off he goes on his grey mare Meg to meet the elements. He eventually come to the Kirk at Alloway where he sees lights and as he looks closer he sees that the coffins in the graveyard are open and the bodies are dancing. Also sitting there is the devil, "auld Nick", watching the activities. Most of the bodies are old and ugly but there is one young lady, wearing a short night dress, a "cutty sark". He watches her and gets so enthusiastic that he gets carried away,

> "And roars out "Weel done Cutty Sark"
> And in an instant all was dark."

Then the problem begins. The whole host of witches chase Tam, who realises that if he can cross water he will be safe. He just makes the cornerstone of the bridge but unfortunately Meg's tail is pulled off. He makes it home, however, to his wife Kate. The final verse of the tale should perhaps be sent out with all GMC literature, just to remind doctors of the evils of drink.

> "now, wha this tale o' truth shall read
> Ilk man and mother's son take heed:
> Whene'er to drink you are inclined,

Or cutty sarks run in your mind,
Think! Ye may buy the joys o'er dear:
Remember Tam O'Shanter's mare."

SOME CONCLUSIONS

First, and perhaps most obviously, each of the books made an excellent re-read and there is real pleasure in re-discovering their language and passion. They were not the only books read over this holiday break, A.S. Byatt's "Possession" being an outstanding additional one, but that's another story. However, they do illustrate the wide range of stories, narratives and tales which can be told and the variety of purposes for which they have been written: for entertainment and enjoyment, for guidance and moral underpinning and teaching and to give a sense of history and culture.

Medical stories are the same. They give depth to the concept of a profession (see Calman 1994, Irvine 1997) and can be entertaining yet educational. They do give a sense of place and of time and meaning for much of the work of the doctor. Telling a good story, also known as the clinical presentation, is partly an art and partly a science. As Chaucer shows, it can be done with humour and attention to detail. Doctors have great practice at telling and listening to stories, as this has been part of being a doctor since before Hippocrates. It is also a privilege.

The books chosen for this holiday interlude reinforce the power and potential of narrative and were great fun to relax with. They illustrate, often with humour, the range of human emotions and feelings and there is still much we can learn from them.

REFERENCES

Bettelheim B, The Uses of Enchantment. 1976. Penguin, Harmondsworth Press,

Calman,K.C. The profession of medicine, 1994 Brit. Med J, 309, 1140-43

Irvine,D. I. Professionalism and self-regulation in a changing world. Brit. Med.J. 314, 1540-2. II, Monitoring good practice, protecting patients from poor performance. Brit. Med.J. 314, 1163-5

Annexe 2
Harold The Dauntless *Sir Walter Scott*

CONCLUSIONS

There is a mood of mind we all have known
On drowsy eye, or dark low'ring day,
When the tired spirits lose their sprightly tone,
And nought can chase the lingering hours away;
Dull on our soul falls Fancy's dazzling ray,
And wisdom holds his steadier torch in vain,
Obscured the painting seems, mistuned the lay,
Nor dare we of our listless load complain,
For who for sympathy may seek that cannot tell of pain?

The jolly sportsman knows such drearihood
When bursts in deluge the autumnal rain,
Clouding that morn which threats the heath-cock's brood;
Of such, in summer's drought, the anglers plain,
Who hope the soft, mild southern shower in vain;
But, more than all, the discontented fair,
Whom father stern and sterner aunt restrain
From county-ball, or race occurring rare,
While all her friends around their vestments gay prepare.

Ennui! or, as our mothers call'd thee, Spleen!
To thee we owe full many a rare device;
Thine is the sheaf of painted cards, I ween,
The rolling billiard-ball, the rattling dice,
The turning-lathe for framing gimcrack nice;
The amateur's blotch'd pallet thou mayst claim,
Retort, and air-pump threatening frogs and mice
(Murders disguised by philosophic name),
And much of trifling grave, and much of buxom game.
Then of the books, to catch thy drowsy glance
Compiled, what bard the catalogue may quote!
Plays, poems, novels, never read but once;-

But not of such the take fair Edgeworth wrote,
That bears thy name, and is thine antidote;
And not of such the strain my Thomson sung,
Delicious dreams inspiring by his note,
What time to Indolence his harp he strung:
Oh! might my lay be rankíd that happier list among!

Each hath his refuge whom thy cares assail.
For me, I love my study-fire to trim
And con right vacantly some idle tale,
Displaying on the couch each listless limb,
Till on the drowsy page the lights grow dim,
And doubtful slumber half supplies the theme,
While antique shapes of knight and giant grim,
Damsel and dwarf, in long procession gleam,
And the romancer's tale becomes the reader's dream.

'Tis thus my malady I well may bear,
Albeit outstretchíd like Pope's own Paridel
Upon the rack of a too-easy chair,
And find, to cheat the time, a powerful spell
In old romaunts of errantry that tell,
Or later legends of the Fairy-folk,
Or Oriental tale of Afrite fell,
Of Genii, Talisman, and broad wing'd Roc,
Though taste may blush and frown,
And sober reason mock.

Oft at such season, too, will rhymes unsought
Arrange themselves in some romantic lay;
The which, as things unfitting graver thought,
Are burnt or blotted on some wiser day
These few survive; and, proudly let me say,
Court not the critic's smile, nor dread his frown;
They well may serve to while an hour away,
Nor does the volume ask for more renown
Than Ennui's yawning smile what time she drops it down.

Printed in the United Kingdom for the Stationery Office
by CW Print, Loughton
TJ 002049 C5 7/00